"Finding One's Self"
in
Sport and Physical Activity

T0208008

Earle F. Zeigler

Ph.D., D.Sc., LL.D., FNAK
The University of Western Ontario
London, Ontario, Canada

Trafford
2012

ISBN: 978-1-4669-6033-6 (sc)
ISBN: 978-1-4669-6034-3 (e)

Library of Congress Control Number: 2012917834

Trafford rev. 09/21/2012

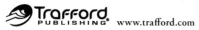 www.trafford.com

North America & international
toll-free: 1 888 232 4444 (USA & Canada)
phone: 250 383 6864 ♦ fax: 812 355 4082

DEDICATION

This book is dedicated to those selfless counselors who over the years have been advising young people as to the various options open to them as they seek a purpose for their lives in a field that can be partially characterized as human physical activity in sport, exercise, play and dance...

Conceptual Index

Dedication   3
Conceptual Index   5
Preface   10

PART 1: INTRODUCTION   16

   1. The Decision to Enter the Field   16
   2. The Role of the Academic Counselor   17
   3. Inadequate Philosophical Orientation   18
   4. The Present Situation   19
   5. The Need to Determine a Professional Philosophy   22
   6. Changes That Are Occurring   24
   7. Where Do We Go from Here?   28
   8. Stages of Philosophical Development   28
   9. Concluding Statement   31

PART 2: CARRYING OUT A SOCIETAL EVALUATION   32

  Where Are You on a Socio-Political Spectrum?
  (A Self-Evaluation for North Americans)   32
   Instructions   32
   Question #1   The United Nations   33
   Question #2   Foreign Aid   35
   Question #3   War and Peace   33
   Question #4   Hostage Crises   35
   Question #5   Protests and Rioting   36
   Question #6   Public Welfare   37
   Question #7   Freedom of Speech and Press   38
   Question #8   Economics and Business   39
   Question #9   Law and Order   41
   Question #10 Population Control   42
   Question #11 Trade Unions   44
   Question #12 Highly Competitive Sport   46
   Question #13 Gay and Lesbian Relationships   47
   Question #14 Environmental Crisis   51
   Question #15 Cloning and Cellular Research   52
  What Was Your Score?   52
  Discussion   56

PART 3: CARRYING OUT A SELF-EVALUATION   57

What Do I Believe?
(A self-evaluation checklist)   57
   Instructions   57
   Category I
   The Nature of Reality (Metaphysics)   58
   Category II
   Ethics and Morality (Axiology/Values)   60
   Category III
   Educational Aims and Objectives   63
   Category IV
   The Educative Process (Epistemology)   65
   Category V
   Values in Recreation Education   68
   Category VI
   Values in Physical Activity Education
   & Educational   71
   Answers   75

   Table 1: Summarizing Tally for Self-Evaluation   76
   Further Instructions   76
   Figure 3: The Freedom-Constraint Spectrum   79

PART 4: GUIDING STUDENTS TO LITERACY
      IN FIELDS ALLIED TO HUMAN
      PHYSICAL ACTIVITY   80

   Definitions   82
   Cultural Literacy   83
   Physical Activity Education   85
   Professional Preparation Development
     for the Physical (Activity) Educator   87
   A Need for Redirection and Rejuvenation   90
   How the Field of "Physical (Activity) Education"
     Should React to the Arrival of
     the Discipline of "Kinesiology"   91
   The Aftermath of a New Name   92
   The Unhappy Plight of Physical Education:

"Good Old 'PE'."   96
Time for Reflection   97
How "PHE" Should React to "Kin"...   98
Looking to the Future   101
A Proposed Taxonomy for the Curriculum
    in Physical Activity Education   101
Table 1: Undergraduate Curriculum in Kinesiology
    & Physical Activity Education   104
The Field Should Develop and Promote
    Its Own Discipline and Its Own Profession   105
An Inventory of Scientific Findings
    About Developmental Physical Activity
    Is Needed Right Now   107
Ordered Principles or Generalizations   107
A Plan Leading Toward an Ever-Expanding
Competencies and Skills Required
    for Professional Literacy   108
A Systems Model for Managerial Effectiveness   111
Competencies and Skills Required for Professional
    Literacy   112
Concluding Statement   119
References   122

PART 5: SHOWING SOCIAL CONCERN
             AS SPORT MANAGEMENT DEVELOPS
             TENABLE THEORY   123

Hard Questions About Present Social Institutions   128
Analyzing Sport's Role in Society   131
Sport Management Theory and Practice   135
Need for a Theory of Sport Management   140
A Proposed Taxonomy for Sport Management   140
Table 2:
Undergraduate Curriculum in Sport Management   141
Figure 1:
A Model for Sport Management Development   143
The Next Step for the
    Sport Management Profession   146
    Formulation of an Inventory of Scientific Findings   150
    How the Inventory Would Be Constructed   153

Concluding Statement   154
References   155

PART 6: MAKING PERSONAL AND GROUP DECISIONS   159

Decision-Making in Sport
and Physical Activity Education
(With an Ethical Dimension When Needed   160
   Recommended Sequential Steps
   in the Decision-Making Process   165
      Part A   166
      Employ three-step approach if the case
      under consideration has ethical considerations
      Part B   166
      Introduce the layout of the argument
      Part C   166
         1) Determination of the main problem after
           consideration of the various sub-problems.
         2) Explication of any knowledge-base.
         3) Analysis of the main problem through
           application of a "three-step ethical
           approach.
         4) Analyze the various personalities and their
           relationships.
         5) Formulation of only those alternative
           solutions to the ethical problem that
           appear to be relevant, possible, and
           meaningful.
         6) Elaboration of the proposed alternative
           solutions
         7) Selection of the preferred alternative
           solution.
         8) Assessment and determination of
           principles/generalizations.
      Appendix:
      A Sample Case: Midwestern University   172

**PART 7: USING A MARKETING ORIENTATION FOR
AN ATHLETIC/RECREATION PROGRAM   183**
(John T. Campbell, M.A.,
Toronto, ON, Canada is co-author)

Introduction   183
Background of the Marketing Orientation Concept 186
Marketing Management for Athletics
      & Physical Recreation   188
Figure 1: Systems Analysis Applied
      to Sport Marketing   189
Concluding Statement   191
Appendix:
Program Evaluation Schedule   193
      Step One Through Step Five   195
Evaluation Schedule Summary   210

**PART 8: EVALUATING THE ADMINISTRATOR
BY FACULTY MEMBERS   213**

Appraisal Guide for the Administrator/Manager
      Instructions (General)   214
      Instructions (Specific)   215
            1. Job Knowledge
            2. Planning and Organizing Work
            3. Supervisory Functions
            4. Working with People
            5. Personal Traits
            6. Drive and Initiative
            8. Cooperation and Team play
General Overall Rating   221

**PART 9: EVALUATING LIFE'S
LEISURE COMPONENT   222**

A Test For Self-Evaluation
Of Your "RQ" (Recreation Quotient   223
      Category 1
      Sports and Physical Activity   224
      Category 2

Social Activities 225
Category 3
Communicative Activities 224
Category 4
Aesthetic & Creative Activities ("Cultural") 226
Category 5
Educational Activities 227
Analysis 228
Recommendations / Suggestions 228

**PART 10: BALANCING LIFE'S CONFLICTING ASPECTS:
A CHALLENGE FOR THE SPORT
AND PHYSICAL ACTIVITY PROFESSIONAL** 231

Introduction 231
A Physical Activity Administrator Should
Understand the Ramifications of Ecology for
Humankind 232
Coordinating Systems Analysis with Human
and Natural Ecologic Interaction in the
the *Organizational* Task of the Administrator 235
Figure 1:
A Systems Model Describing Human Ecologic
Interaction for the Manager of Sport
and Physical Activity 237
Figure 2:
A Schematic Model for the Administrative Process
That Embodies a Systems Approach 240
Figure 3:
A Systems Analysis Model for Managerial
Effectiveness of a Professional Program
for Physical Activity Administration 243
Coordinating Systems Analysis with Human
and Natural Ecologic Interaction in the
Personal Development of the Administrator 243
Merging the Two Approaches to Achieve
Both: A Successful *Professional* Life and
a Personally Fulfilling Life 246
Conclusion 247
References 248

PREFACE

In this book I draw on many aspects of my 70 years of experience with the field of physical activity education (including sport) to offer some advice to the student's academic counselor, as well as to the young person either considering entry into a professional- or disciplinary-degree program in either kinesiology and physical activity education *or in sport management*. The book would also be useful to a person just starting out as a young professional relating to these related areas of study.

It would be a rare week that went by (prior to semi-retirement) when I did not talk to at least one young man or woman about his or her future in the field that involves human physical activity in one or more ways. As an academic counselor, my task was typically to explain to this young man or young woman in a few well-chosen words that the field of human physical activity overall is much more than simply a teacher, a coach, a teacher/coach, a fitness specialist, a professor and/or administrator in a college or university, a sport manager or sport columnist–or even a performer of selected physical skills (i.e., a professional athlete)–as important a task as any of these areas can be.

It is also true that an outstanding athlete who specializes in physical activity education-kinesiology to understand his or her performance better–or at times because the person might think it would be easier and thus provide more time for actual participation in sport! To give specific advice is difficult, and I was not always certain just how much to say. I didn't want to bore this young person with my experiences in the various aspects of the field–or even "turn him off…" Actually so much depended on the young man's or woman's prior experiences and innate intellectual ability.

I usually told them about both the advantages and disadvantages, emphasizing the former more than the latter. Then I typically concluded by stating that, even though there is overcrowding in some areas within the profession of education or the discipline of kinesiology, there always seems to be room for a well-qualified, conscientious, devoted professional person striving to improve the level of developmental physical activity within people's lives–or even in his/her own life for that matter. As he or she left, I also told this young person to keep in touch and not to hesitate to contact me or one of my associates if a problem arose. Finally, I wished the young man or woman good luck.

However, after the student left, I began to wonder if I had said and done the right things. Of course, perhaps nothing I could have said or done would have changed his or her thinking radically. I hoped sincerely that the university experience was such that this typical professional student would emerge upon graduation as a competent teacher/coach of sport and physical activity education, a sport manager ready to assume professional leadership of the highest type, or a scholar researcher in higher education.

What then happens to this young person? Many influences affect his or her development, both good and bad. Eventually the student acquires certain knowledge, competencies, and skills. He may have been a good student, a fair student, or a poor student. Rarely is this person, male or female, either an outstanding student or an outstanding athlete. However, there are the all-to-few exceptions (!). In addition, along the way the individual develops a set of attitudes (speaking psychologically). I must add that too infrequently does this young man or woman show an inclination after graduation to be really active in at least one professional or scholarly society. Then I wonder where she or he went wrong-or where we failed as counselors or teachers...

After the introductory phase of the book (Part 1), a number of basic topics will be considered in the ordered listed below: Initially, in Part 2, the student/advisee is asked to get involved with a self-evaluation questionnaire concerning his/her socio-political beliefs (e.g., (freedom of speech and press, environmental crisis, war and peace). This is followed (Part 3) by an explanation of the need for *truly basic self-evaluation* with the introduction of a checklist for the prospective professional (i.e., teacher/coach/manager/scholar/"whatever") to complete. This involves educational aims and objectives, the educative process, ethics, etc..

In Part 4 the student is asked to consider what it is, at this point, that he/she believes he really wants out of life. At this point the question is in regard to the way he/she looks at future employment. Is employment going to be "a job", "a trade". "a profession", or "a mission in life" Obviously, this gradation presented here as to response to this query is tremendously important. Does the student want to be a teacher, a teacher/coach, a sport manager, a scholar or scientist, or in some cases even has the inherent ability and skill to be a professional performer.

Next in Part 5 the prospective teacher/coach/manager is introduced to an approach for decision-making in sport and physical activity education through the introduction of a case method technique where detailed analysis might occur (including the possibility of an ethical dimension being added when needed).

Then in sequential order, Part 6 discusses the question of employment of strategic market planning to assess what progress has been made in the management of a program of sport and physical recreation. The steps recommended range from definition of the organization to employment of a pre-determined marketing mix as the organization moves toward achievement of its goals.

Penultimately, in Part 7, the subject of administrator evaluation by faculty members in a program is presented through use of an appraisal guide whereby those serving under the leadership of the manager, for example, are provided with an opportunity to assess his/her leadership based on the various dimensions of the task.

Finally, the professional person is offered a test for self-evaluation of his/her "RQ" or recreation quotient to determine whether he/she understand what "the good life" might hold in store.. All in all, these self-testing, evaluative devices and quizzes and the subsequent discussion could be most helpful to the young professional entering the field in this new 21st century.

The field of physical (activity) education, and the variations thereof involved with human physical activity in sport, exercise, or some form of expressive movement, has had a history of about 150 years. For example, in 1861 in the United States a private academy began to train teachers of exercise and related physical activity for both schools and society at large. Then, people started earning money for sport performance. Next many colleges and universities began to hire men and women as professors to teach undergraduate and graduate students for employment as teachers of physical education (and later as coaches) in public and private schools.

After World War I, professors in these same universities began to undertake scholarly endeavor and research borrowing knowledge and techniques from the natural sciences, social sciences, and humanities. Then, about 40 years ago, as a number of students began to show interest in becoming sport managers-not physical activity educators or coaches-of some type in the public or private sector, gradually a number of distinct professional preparation programs began to prepare sport managers along the lines of those training physical educators.

When people would ask me what the future held for them within this multifaceted field within education or as a profession in the public sector, all that I could say is that it was a "judgment call". I said this because the "path to the top" was unclear depending upon the direction taken, the talents possessed, and the zeal displayed. I would typically reply that basically they held their future–and that of the overall field of human physical activity in sport, dance, play, and exercise actually–in their own hands. And yet such "possession" was to a limited extent. I still believe, what we make it–except for the unforeseen whims of fate. Life is largely what we are able to make out of it.

This is a rough analysis of the role I played as one academic counselor at both the undergraduate and graduate levels in physical activity education, kinesiology, and sport management at three universities from 1949 to 1989 (i.e., Western Ontario, Michigan, Illinois, and then Western Ontario again). (I taught and coached ay Yale University in the 1940s, but there was no professional preparation program there.)

As I look back at what I went through with the various stages of professional preparation and professional preparation, I now can appreciate what a "catch-as-catch-can" routine it was. This is especially true since I started out–after a brief stint as an unprepared YMCA physical education secretary seeking also to become prepared to be a professor of German. I believe the transition from one stage to another could have been so much better, so much smoother. This is why, at this very late stage of life, I decided to review the situation (i.e., what I went through and discovered) with an eye to possibly making the reader's transition and progress so much smoother than mine was. Bon voyage...

Earle F. Zeigler, 2012

PART 1: INTRODUCTION

The Decision to Enter the Field

I often stated that we who entered this field simply made a "judgment call"...

> (Note: By the phrase "entering the field", I mean the field of human physical activity either within public or private education as an educator, or in the public sector as a professional practitioner. The field/profession is necessarily under girded by a discipline that is becoming known as kinesiology in North America)

Such words may still today smack of a (non-philosophic) *idealism* that we, in more pessimistic moments, view as out of date. Today the average student specializing in physical activity education generally, or in some area of specialization within it, is typically *realistic* (speaking non-philosophically again) and often quite materialistic as well. Many young people contemplating this future in the field probably made this decision initially on the basis of athletic experience with a high school or university coach. The young person admired the coach greatly, and from that point assessed his or her own personal athletic and intellectual ability that probably included a sociable nature and a liking of people. Then, often against the presumably better judgment of parents–especially if they were so-called middle class–a decision was made to be a physical activity educator, a coach, a sport manager, a professional athlete, or "whatever"–such whatever" being *somehow* related to the overall field.

Even today, if a male, this young man may see himself coaching a successful high school football or basketball team, and then possibly going on to presumably "bigger and better things" as a college or university coach. Or today he/she may have been intrigued by the expanding area of sport and physical activity management and decide that this is where a life purpose can be found. Still further, some young people who specialize in sport and physical activity because of their *innate* physical ability go on to earn very high incomes as professional athletes. Less frequently young people choose our profession initially because of a desire to help "normal" and "special" people become "physical activity & health educated," so to speak.

The Role of the Academic Counselor

As an academic counselor, my task was typically to explain to this young man or young woman in a few well-chosen words that the field of developmental physical activity overall is much more than simply being an athletic coach or a sport manager or a physical activity education teacher–as important a task as either of these three areas can be. It is also true that an outstanding athlete who specializes in physical activity education-kinesiology to understand his or her performance better–or at times because the person might think it would be easier and thus provide more time for actual participation in sport! To give specific advice is difficult, and I was not always certain just how much to say. I didn't want to bore this young person with my experiences in the various aspects of the field–or even "turn him off... Actually so much depended on the young man's or woman's prior experiences and innate intellectual physical or mental ability.

I usually told them about both the advantages and disadvantages, emphasizing the former more than the latter. Then I typically concluded by stating that, even though there is overcrowding in some areas within the profession, there always seems to be room for a well-qualified, conscientious, devoted professional person striving to improve the level of developmental physical activity within people's lives–or in his/her own life for that matter. As he or she left, I also told this young person to keep in touch and not to hesitate to contact me if a problem arose. Finally, I wished the young man or woman good luck.

However, after the student left, I began to wonder if I had said and done the right things. Of course, perhaps nothing I could have said or done would have changed his or her thinking radically. I hoped sincerely, of course that the university experience was such that this typical professional student would emerge upon graduation as a competent teacher/coach of sport and physical activity education, sport manager ready to assume professional leadership of the highest type, or scholar researcher in higher education.

What then happens to this young person? Many influences affect his or her development, both good and bad. Eventually the student acquires certain knowledge, competencies, and skills. He may have been a good student, a fair student, or a poor student. Rarely is this person, male or female, either an outstanding student or an outstanding athlete. However, there are the all-to-few exceptions (!). In addition, along the way the individual develops a set of attitudes (speaking psychologically). I must add that too infrequently does this young man or woman show an inclination after graduation to be really active in one or more professional or scholarly organizations. Then I wonder where she or he went wrong-or where perhaps we failed as counselors or teachers. . . .

Inadequate Philosophical Orientation

A great many people have philosophical beliefs, but in the present world situation they are terribly vague about them. Unfortunately the average person still thinks of philosophy as something that is beyond his or her capability–a most difficult intellectual activity. This may be true in the case of the trained professional philosopher who functions in the present scholarly approach to the discipline, but it should not be true in the realm of applied philosophy where more ordinary mortals must come to grips with daily life.

Having been frightened by the presumed complexity of all philosophical endeavor, the average person struggles along with an implicit philosophy based on personal experience. When problems arise, decisions are typically based on common sense. This isn't necessarily bad, but it could be a lot better. The deliberate, conscious development of a philosophy would help people fashion a better world for the future. It should be a considered position based on the past and the ongoing scientific discoveries of the present. Without philosophic thought we can never know if we have reasoned reasonably correctly about our goals in life. Some may ask immediately whether science might not achieve this for us by its everlasting probing into the unknown characteristically activated by an endless stream of emerging hypotheses. The answer to this question, I believe, rests with a correct understanding of the relationship between philosophy and science.

My position is that philosophy should be infinitely more than a handmaiden to science, as important a function as the former may be. Both are most interested in knowledge; they ask questions and want answers. Scientific investigators turn in facts; the philosopher must be cognizant of these advances. However, my ongoing belief is that the major function of philosophy starts where science leaves off by attempting to synthesize. What do all of these scientific findings mean? When you become concerned about the ultimate meaning of these facts, then you are attempting to philosophize in the best sense.

The Present Situation

I found that the large majority of educators in kinesiology and physical activity education or in sport and physical activity management haven't had the opportunity, or haven't taken the time, to work out their personal philosophies. They arrive at an implicit philosophy of life naturally in the course of their maturation, but only rarely has such a philosophic stance been worked out rationally with care and concern. Granted, along the way there may have been a great deal of discussion about aims and objectives, but it has usually been carried out in bits and pieces in each and every course in helter-skelter fashion. The usual result is that students want no more of it. They are anxious to learn the much more tangible competencies and skills that they can use on the job. And so they leave us as graduates not *really* knowing why they are doing anything and where they are going.

Undergraduates in physical activity education and/or sport management need exactly the same sort of liberal arts and science background in the first two years of the undergraduate curriculum as any person preparing for any profession. The former are needed to develop further the knowledge, skills and competencies of the humanities, social sciences, and natural sciences.

Individuals striving to function intelligently in society need a comprehensive understanding of the historical foundations of our society. They will then be able to study and to appreciate more fully the historical backgrounds of their later-chosen field and the persistent problems that have been faced at the various levels of society through the ages

Years three and four of higher education should be significantly different. More intensive knowledge and competencies in the social sciences should be introduced in years three and four in applied management theory and practice for those wishing to specialize in sport and physical activity management per se. Conversely, the physical activity education–kinesiology major will necessarily spend more time with so-called *hard* science and the subsequent applied aspects of these subjects. Both types of specialization should have an under girding socio-cultural orientation.

Fundamentally, a professional person needs a philosophy of life and/or religion. Furthermore, physical activity education professionals-whether employed in the educational system or in society at large, and/or serving as future parents, should have a philosophy of education in harmony with their philosophy of life. Philosophy of education courses are often available as an elective, but our students usually avoid them because this departmental philosophy to a large degree eventually aped the esoteric analytic approach of the mother discipline (philosophy).

The culmination of this recommended curricular sequence (prior to one theoretically based course in management for physical activity educators and more extensive management training for the embryonic sport manager) should be an outstanding core course experience in sport and physical activity education philosophy, a course in which the young professional begins to develop a personal philosophy relating to his or her specialized field. The hope (the goal!) is that the basic beliefs within the specialized field will be reasonably in harmony with the beliefs about life/religion/education. *Of course, the achievement of a "total" philosophy may well become a lifelong task. The reflective thinking required to accomplish this task, however, is a cheap price to pay for a well-ordered life.*

We have only to look at present programs with their shifting emphases to realize that we are, to quite a degree, vacillating practitioners. This is true for us in physical activity education whether related to educational institutions, and it is also true for most practitioners in our allied professions as well. The situation in sport management appears somewhat different where success is related more to economic achievement. Why is such vacillation happening? I believe this is so because even most of our experienced leaders have not worked out personal philosophies that are consistent and logical in their various phases! So where does that leave the rest of us?

When a person becomes a member of an established profession (e.g., education, management), we assume that he or she will exert some leadership in this line of endeavor. We should be able to expect that this individual possesses at least some of the "basic building blocks" required to establish what might be called a life purpose. Is this too much to ask? Evidently it is, because even many of our leaders become hazy when asked to express a philosophy. To be sure, they have a lot of opinions, isolated and often basically contradictory. It's a little like saying, "I'm for good and against sin." The difficulty comes when we are asked to define what's good and what's bad, or what is right action and what would be wrong.

Where does physical activity education and related health considerations fit into life's picture today? Actually, I like to define our field of endeavor as "developmental physical activity in exercise, sport, and related expressive movement for normal, accelerated, and special populations throughout life." What does this consist of? Why it is it needed? What does it do to a child, a young person, an adult, an older man or woman? To what extent can we prove that it does what we say it does? What will its future be? What could its future be? What should its future be?

The Need to Determine a Professional Philosophy

The time has arrived when the true educator in physical activity education or the enlightened sport manager should adopt a basic personal philosophy. Science, whether "natural" or "social", and philosophy have complementary roles to play in aiding the field to find its place in society. For too long we have ignored the wisdom of these branches of learning in carrying out our professional endeavor. Lately, there has been an increased interest in science with a corresponding loss of interest in philosophy.

Philosophy, approached normatively, can help us attack the basic problems of the physical activity education field or the sport management specialization in a systematic fashion. In the first place, philosophy will enable the prospective professional a developmental physical activity educator Except for students majoring in sport and physical education in Catholic universities, our professional students rarely, if ever, take an introductory course in philosophy or in the philosophy of religion to view the profession as a whole. He or she will not see the professional task as that of an exercise teacher, an athletic coach, or a special education teacher. In this sense, philosophy would be a criticism of experience.

Philosophy will help the physical activity educator, for example, to fashion for himself or herself a mental image of what his field physical *ought to be* in the light of a personal philosophy of developmental physical activity with a life pattern. This mental image (or philosophic stance) will be prospective in the sense that it will form a vanguard leading practice in the field. It is true that there will be conflicting philosophies. However, at least people will be reasonably logical and consistent in their approaches no matter which philosophic stance they accept.

A professional educator's philosophy of physical activity education-one adopted by consensus on the field's values and norms-would eventually have to be practical, or it would soon become worthless in the eyes of many. An instrumental philosophy would necessarily imitate science in part, but it would serve only as an initial plan for action. What this means is that science can describe physical activity education as it is; philosophy can help to picture it as it should be. The same can be said for the allied fields-for any professional endeavor for that matter. In addition, philosophy can fill in for science temporarily, since its method and techniques are faster.

A philosophy of developmental physical activity as it relates to physical activity education undoubtedly has a relationship to the general field of philosophy. However, there are varied and conflicting views on this point. Most obvious is that which holds a philosophy of life basic and primary to any so-called departmental philosophy (e.g., educational philosophy, physical activity education philosophy). To the mother discipline-to the extent that one of several traditional positions is held (e.g., idealism, realism)- is assigned the establishment of fundamental principles. Pragmatism, of course, doesn't start with immutable, fundamental principles; here a value is that fact which, when applied to a life situation, becomes useful. Thus, the ongoing dilemma for the pragmatist is to decide which value or values will help achieve life's purposes in the best way. Both values and goals may well be held only temporarily as life evolves. An analytic philosophic approach or an existential-phenomenological orientation are other approaches that may be taken.

My position over the years has been one in which I hold a "live and let live" attitude with students. In my opinion no effort should be made to indoctrinate a student in one direction or another. However, I believe strongly that a young professional educator ought to consider carefully that which is available: In other words, whether philosophically he or she has a largely progressivistic (liberal), essentialistic (traditional), existential-phenomenological, or analytic orientation. At the least, physical activity educators should be able to determine for themselves under which "banner" they stand. At present many professionals are dilettantes and hence present no solid arguments for many of the beliefs they may hold. We should at least know which side of the fence we are on-or even whether we are sitting on the fence! Whatever one's position may be, a decision can be made whether to stay there when dark clouds threaten.

Today there are many serious problems and conflicts dangerously splitting the human physical activity field. Some say there is no such thing as *physical* education, for example. (They are correct!) Others say that it's sport that it's all about. Still others argue that physical fitness is our primary task, and that we should be about our business and forget the whole idea of concomitant learning. Further, to what extent do we (or should we) have a responsibility for so-called special physical activity or adapted programs for children and youth with special needs?

It can be argued that the serious problems we are facing are only signs that the field is undergoing modification. By this I mean that we are now definitely tending to restrict, limit, or qualify what it is that *we*-in what I am terming *physical activity education*-should be doing professionally. This is an optimistic outlook, however; and it can be argued conversely that many of these problems or changes are being forced upon us because we have for too long sought to be "all things to all people" or "jacks of all trades, masters of none." Whatever the case may be, we have indubitably reached the point in our development as educators where we must sharpen our focus. My fear, however, is that this process of modification-from whichever direction the thrust toward change is coming-is occurring too slowly. In the meantime, additional social forces are crowding us, are limiting us in various undesirable ways, and in the process are often buffeting us unmercifully.

Changes That Are Occurring

As I see it, the following are some of the changes that are occurring:

> 1. Because in the past the field of physical activity education has sought to be "all things to all people," *we now don't know exactly what we stand for.* Soon we won't be certain whether push-ups and jogging still belong to us. What ever happened to Arthur Steinhaus' "principal principles" of physical education? Where does our major thrust lie?

2. *All sorts of name changes are occurring* to explain either what people think we are doing or should be doing, not to mention how they can camouflage the unsavory connotation of the term "physical education." Thus, we are becoming kinesiology, human kinetics, exercise science, ergonomics, sport management, sport studies, kinanthropology, or what have you?

3. The advent of Sputnik; the subsequent "race for the moon" and how this affected education, science, and technology; Conant's devastating criticism of the presumed academic content of our curricula in the early 1960s; and the subsequent, almost frantic, drive for a body of knowledge for the field placed us in a curious position as a-*we really don't know where or what our body of knowledge is*. Nowhere is it available to us in a series of ordered principles or generalizations based on an accepted taxonomy of sub–disciplinary and sub–professional specializations.

4. *We are not supporting our professional organizations anywhere nearly sufficiently* either at the state or provincial, district in the United States, or national levels in either the United States or Canada. As a result, they are struggling with insufficient funding and thereby are incapable of meeting the many demands being made by the practitioners.

5. A corollary of No. 4 is that *an ever-widening gap is developing* between what might be called the related-discipline sport societies and the established field of physical education within education. For example, we find the North American Society for the Sociology of Sport, the International Association for the Philosophy of Sport (formerly the PSSS), The Association for the (Anthropological) Study of Play, the North American Society for Sport History, the American College of Sport Medicine, and many others who could care less, to put it bluntly, what happens to the field of physical

activity education (as defined by the National Association for Sport and Physical Education (NASPE in the U.S.A.) and PHE Canada (formerly the Canadian Association for Health, Physical Education and Recreation or CAHPER in Canada). An interesting fact is that most of these latter-day societies and organizations might well flounder overnight if those people paid by physical education departments were to suddenly disappear from their membership rosters.

6. Despite the fact that the College Entrance Examination Board or CEEB in the United States in the early 1970s established a commission that eventually *recommended much greater weight and consideration in entrance requirements be allotted to certain important qualities and attributes over and above the traditional verbal factor and mathematical factor* (e.g., sensitivity and commitment to social responsibility, political and social leadership, ability to adapt to new situations), there is no evidence that we have stressed, or even understand to any degree, whether physical activity education/kinesiology majors possess originally or subsequently achieve knowledge, competence, or skill in any of the total of nine vital components as recommended by the CEEB. In Canada there never was any question in this regard: the academic average is still the one deciding factor in decision-making in regard to university entrance, and in Ontario (for example) there is talk of bringing back provincial-level examinations.

7. *Another unacceptable series of gaps* has developed among the people in physical activity education concerned with the bioscience aspects of the field; those investigating the social science and humanities aspects of the discipline; a third group concerned with the professional preparation of physical educators and with investigation concerning what might be call the sub-professional aspects of the field (e.g., curriculum, instructional methodology, supervision, management);

and the professional practitioners in the field where divisions often exist among the physical activity educator, the coach, and the dance person.

8. *A further disturbing development took place.* For several reasons, at least one of which is our own fault, the highly influential and volatile area of competitive sport has become a playground for several of our allied professions, as well as for an increasing number of people in what we call our related disciplines. Here I am referring to the close identification of the recreation profession with highly competitive sport and fitness, the interest of health educators with exercise science, the involvement of physiotherapists in adaptive or special physical education, the developing relationship between business administration and intercollegiate sport, and, of course, the gradually awakening interest of historians, philosophers, sociologists, psychologists, anthropologists, physiologists, medical professors, biomechanics specialists, etc. in competitive sport.

9. Steadily, because physical activity education has been struggling to acquire an "academic image" since it was criticized so sharply by Conant way back in 1963, *a larger wedge than ever has been driven between physical education and intercollegiate athletics.* (Of course, that small but highly visible segment of intercollegiate sport that may be called "big-time, commercial, intercollegiate athletics" has been subject to all sorts of abuses throughout this century.) This has been a most unfortunate development for us and for them, too. A small group of pressure-driven administrators and coaches has used us and many of their colleagues in other disciplines as well, not to mention the unethical way in which many so-called scholar-athletes have been sacrificed along the way (e.g., the very large percentage of black athletes who have not graduated). This has been most unfortunate for all concerned.

10. Finally, and it is odd that listing such as this always seem to include 10 items, *I detect an uneasiness or malaise no doubt brought on by the developments of the past years.* It is quite possible that the most crucial aspect of the modification that I claim we are undergoing is typified by so many people who seem ready and willing to write off physical activity education. There is evidence that many within the field are losing their will to win. In the final analysis this aspect of the modification I have been describing could be the most devastating of all the aspects of modification indicated above.

Where Do We Go from Here?

Looking to the future, it is quite possible that there are still other problems that are also preventing the profession (s?) from presenting a united, determined, and powerful front at a time when the worth of our programs in society generally, as well as within the educational picture, is being challenged continuously. For example, if we can find agreement on the centrality of "beneficial physical activity" in programs furthering physical activity education, kinesiology, and sport management, we will all be "working on the same side of the street"! The answers to the questions, and the solutions to the problems, cannot be provided by the uninformed or the misinformed. The highest type of reflective thinking is needed. A personal stand can come only through the development of a consistent physical activity education philosophy that includes sport and its wise management.

Stages of Philosophical Development

I close Part 1 with my belief that a professional person may indeed go through five stages of philosophic development as follows:

1. *Ostrich Stage.* He may find that he have been in the *ostrich stage* up to now. He may have buried his head in the sand (as this bird is reported to do periodically) and

refused to allow himself to become aware of the conflicting philosophies that exist in the world, in the culture, or within his approach to the field promoting beneficial physical activity.

2. *Cafeteria Stage.* Or perhaps she may have climbed the ladder (in this instance a *five-rung stepladder*) a bit further and are at the *cafeteria stage*. This involves selecting "some of this and some of that" which looks appetizing for one's philosophical fare. This eclectic approach has a great deal of appeal initially, but there appears to be strong evidence that it is generally regarded as philosophically indefensible. It may, of course, merely be one stage in an individual's development, but it is to be hoped that the devoted professional will soon make her way higher on the ladder.

In assessing *eclecticism*, Wegener in the mid-1950s saw it as "a mosaic of diverse conceptions rather than a genuine integration of thought." He called it a "mixture" which he hoped would become a compound (p. 31). As I see it, there is every reason to believe that a person will be attracted by certain elements of the various approaches. The fear I have is that a person may lift something out of context and insert it somewhere else where it simply does not belong. Thus I see this second stage simply as a resting place along the way up the ladder. If a person does not proceed higher into more rarefied air, I think he or she risks not achieving one's professional potential in the final analysis. (This goes back to my longstanding argument that a fine professional person should become a "missionary" for the promotion of the profession.)

3. *Fence-Sitter Stage.* The third rung of the ladder is a popular place. This rung has to be a strong one to hold all the people who have gotten this far and no further. I have designated this as the *fence-sitter stage* or level. Here we find people who have matured a bit more and

have found, perhaps unconsciously to a degree, that they are inclining in one philosophic direction or another (e.g. to the left rather than the right; perhaps toward an existential-phenomenological orientation as opposed to a group-oriented position). But beyond that they are unwilling to go. Why? Maybe they're too lazy intellectually, if such a distinction may be made. Perhaps they're vaguely afraid of the consequences of a determined stand. We are told that all too many people are still inclined to be "organization men or women" who don't wish to rock the boat for fear of the possible consequences. Then again, there are often other reasons not disclosed. The late Princeton philosopher, Kaufmann (1973, Chap. 1), coined the term *decidophobia* for a person's fear of autonomy and/or decision-making.

4. *Stage of Early Maturity*. In time I fervently hope that my present advisee (s0 will at least rise to the fourth rung on this proposed philosophical ladder. This I call the *stage of early maturity*. At this point the individual professional has wrestled with herself or himself and the immediate social environment. This person has achieved a quality of unity or harmony that is characteristic of a philosophical position or stance that is reasonably logical or consistent in its various departments. She, if this is the case, is able to justify her convictions (which may earlier have been only tentative persuasions) intellectually to the extent that scientific knowledge, and perhaps faith, can assist her. As a result she has developed strong attitudes that are reflected in the moral ardor of her personal and professional life. It is probably not necessary to say that there is plenty of room on this rung of the ladder. Beware of the strong possibility of intolerance and fanaticism at this point!

5. *Stage of Philosophical Maturity*. As a professional person matures still further, I hope that he/she will gradually achieve wisdom as well as mere knowledge.

If he does, he may arrive at the *stage of philosophical maturity*. This level of personal and professional development can come from a broad and sound experience, diligent study, and ordered reflection. It is at this point that we as individuals realize the supreme importance and need for a certain amount of agreement or consensus on a nation-wide, indeed on a *worldwide*, basis.

Concluding Statement

Thus, no matter which stage of philosophical development a young man or woman may have achieved presently, he may find it necessary periodically based on experience to retrace his/her steps before a personal philosophy emerges that is logical, consistent, and systematic. Obviously there is no hard and fast progression to which a professional person must adhere.

Finally, encourage your advisee to view the journey as a lifelong quest. He or she simply can't go wrong if he goes about it honestly, sincerely, and diligently. People of all ages are searching for meaningful values in their lives. If your advisee as a potential physical activity educator, coach, scholar, researcher, or sport manager (whatever!) can reach his/her life goal, you yourself as academic counselor will also have attained the highest of professional goals as an educator.

PART 2: SOCIETAL EVALUATION

Subsequently I found in the process of developing my course in physical activity education with undergraduates (and with graduate students too from other universities for that matter) that the uncertainty and indecision present in their personal philosophic and/or religious beliefs extended to their socio-political understanding as well. It did seem to me that reasonable consistency—insofar as both general and specific issues were concerned—ought to exist between thoughts and stances taken in both realms. (Of course, I was careful not to influence them unduly on what might be considered their personal "religious positions" assumed. However, I did think it fair to point out inconsistencies as they occurred.)

Where Are You on a Socio-Political Spectrum?
(A Self-Evaluative Questionnaire for North Americans)

by
Earle F. Zeigler, Ph.D.

Instructions:

What really is your socio-political stance or position? This questionnaire will help you figure out where you stand on a socio-political spectrum--not where you may nominally think that you are. When someone asks, "Are you conservative or liberal?" What do you say in response? How can you justify such an answer?

> (Note: Keep in mind that these responses do not necessarily equate with the presently stated platforms of existing political parties in either the United States or Canada.)

Some people will admit that they are radical or reactionary (i.e., far left or far right). Even if you are neutral, or middle-of-the-road, it should be possible to make that determination with his questionnaire. Why is this important? Simply because a person with an "ordered mind" ought to be able to state his/her beliefs and opinions with reasonable consistency based on a set of generally accepted values.

Answer the following questions to the best of your ability in accordance with your reason and/or conscience. You are designating HOW YOU WANT IT TO BE! Where possible, a position has been carefully worded to represent one of the following six positions: (1) REACTIONARY, (2) CONSERVATIVE, (3) MODERATE CONSERVATIVE, (4) MODERATE LIBERAL, (5) LIBERAL, AND (6) RADICAL. In some cases allowing only two options for response (i.e., agreement or disagreement) was deemed best.

On any given question or issue, one's position to the right or left on a spectrum would fluctuate between +3 and +1 or between -3 and -1. When you are finished with the self-evaluation device (i.e. the scores are totaled), it should be possible for you to designate yourself one way or the other. Or perhaps you may be an eclectic (i.e., a person with widely distributed with responses from both sides of the spectrum). Or perhaps you will be a truly middle-of-the-road person (i.e., generally neutral on most questions).

In each question, therefore, please select the answer that comes the closest to reflecting your belief or position as to how you would like that issue to be (!) (Note: The answers have been purposely arranged so that you can't detect a "patterned sequence" each time with a particular question.)

Please encircle the letter (a, b, etc.) that appears before the answer that you select. The scoring system, and a few comments of a explanatory nature about those espousing answers in one category or another are included at the end of the questionnaire.

Question #1 THE UNITED NATIONS

The place of the United Nations in world government should be:

   a. NEGLIGIBLE--i.e., advisory only or possibly eliminated.

   b. MINOR--and used for voluntary arbitration of

international disputes only.

     c. AS AT PRESENT--with members of Council having veto power.

     d. ENLARGED SOMEWHAT--and characterized by more adequate enforcement of decisions.

     e. EXPANDED CONSIDERABLY--and involved with actual enforcement of peacekeeping.

     f. EXPANDED GREATLY--and hold the leading position in world government (a similar relationship as a federal government does to its states or provinces.

Question #2 FOREIGN AID.

     North Americans should:

     a. Stop all foreign aid except when serious natural disasters occur.

     b. Help friendly nations and/or neutral nations strengthen themselves against communistic and similar undemocratic nations by providing economic and educational assistance.

     c. Provide aid to developing nations to the best of our ability, but only to those who ask for such aid and are willing to use it for sound economic development. The channeling of aid through an international agency is basic.

     d. Keep foreign aid to a minimum, getting involved only when it is clearly in our self-interest.

     e. Provide assistance only to free and/or neutral nations.

     f. Aid economically any needy country that requests such help for basic services.

Question #3 WAR AND PEACE.

In regard to military affairs and defense, North Americans should:

a. Work to outlaw war through unilateral disarmament by all nations.

b. Intervene militarily only when required (by United Nations and NATO) and when the need is extreme--and then only in an effort to bring peace and to protect further loss of life. Major powers should disarm to an "irreducible minimum."

c. Give military assistance to free or neutral nations when they request it. Encourage the idea of disarmament.

d. Help friendly and/or neutral nations with military assistance against infiltration by undemocratic ideologies (e.g., communism).

e. Stand prepared to protect the free world and "third world" nations with military forces at all times.

f. Deal ruthlessly with naked aggression wherever it occurs (including use of nuclear power).

Question #4 HOSTAGE CRISES.

Any hostage crisis where one country holds North American citizens at ransom (or for whatever purpose) warrants the following action:

a. An urgent request for an explanation, assurance of safe release, and reparation for damages at the first possible moment.

b. Armed invasion as soon as it becomes apparent that the hostages taken are in danger and will not be released.

c. A protest through diplomatic channels for an explanation with a plea for swift action and the safety of the hostages.

d.   An immediate warning that such kidnapping and terrorist activity will not be tolerated. The foreign government concerned should understand that some direct action will be taken if hostages are not released by a specified date.

e.   The immediate establishment of a naval blockade to the extent possible along with the implementation of other sanctions possible (e.g., freezing of assets).

f.   A sharp protest through diplomatic channels indicating that consideration will be given to what measures might be taken to effect the release of the hostages.

Question #5 PROTESTS AND RIOTING.

Youth, both at home and abroad, are causing considerable concern to governmental officials at all levels. I feel that young people:

a.   Must be made to respect law and order. Rioters who loot should be warned and then shot if they don't stop. Foreign nationals, immigrants, and other marginal persons in these groups should be rooted out, jailed, and/or deported.

b.   Are, in many cases, attempting to move positively toward and improved national and international order. They should be given many different types of roles to play, as well as opportunities to improve the situation through involvement.

c.   Are concerned and need positive leadership from adults who have experience and know-how in such matters. Only a small percentage of these activists are radical and need truly firm control.

d.   Are justified in their struggle to change the basic nature of the society. Ethnic minority groups, Blacks (in the States), and young people should not have to wait forever for much- needed change. Many fundamental institutions must be rebuilt from the ground up.

e. Are proving in many cases to be ungrateful brats. Lax and frightened adults have allowed them to get out of hand too often. Strong adult leadership is required.

f. Are troubled and need guidance from qualified personnel. Only a relatively few are real troublemakers who need to be curbed by force. The large majority of youth will turn out to be decent, law-abiding adults.

Question #6 PUBLIC WELFARE.

Public welfare programs in North America are:

a. Urgently needed and should be coordinated by the federal government. There should be a guaranteed annual income for all needy families sufficient to provide a reasonable standard of living pro-rated to the cost-of-living in the geographical region involved. Billions are needed soon as possible to upgrade all aspects of the lives of the poor and neglected members of society.

b. Best left to states and local governments to provide only the most needy with some assistance. Heads of families (or close relatives) should work to provide for the welfare of their families (and/or close relatives). Government handouts should be kept to an absolute minimum.

c. Needed on a limited basis from all levels of government, but experience has shown that the federal government should set and enforce national standards. In this way all families will have sufficient resources to maintain at least a minimum standard of living. Current disincentives to work must somehow be removed.

d. Unfortunately necessary. Somehow the current disincentives toward work must be eliminated. All male and female recipients should be worked back into the job force--even if doing public service work for their welfare payments. Perhaps by introducing national or regional standards that take into consideration cost of living indexes in the various "high" welfare states.

e. Positively dangerous to the future of our democratic societies on the continent because they are inexorably bringing about a decay of moral fiber. Our North American culture is based on people working for a living. We must become more firm. If those currently on the dole get hungry enough, they'll find some work to do to support themselves and their families.

f. A sop to mislead the poor and trick them into acceptance of the capitalist system. The nation's wealth should be redistributed so as to assure virtual   equality for all people who are willing to be gainfully employed citizens. The current systematic degradation and exploitation of the poor must stop.

Question #7 FREEDOM OF SPEECH AND PRESS.

The rights of freedom of speech and press contained, for example, in the First Amendment of the U.S. Constitution:

a. Are a part of the heritage of free men and women on this continent, but subversive and immoral elements have been allowed to take advantage of these rights. These people and certain social influences threaten to   destroy the fabric of freedom.

b. Are a vital part of the U.S.A.'s and Canada's heritage. We all profit from new and different ideas. However, it is necessary to limit speech and action that present a "clear and present danger" to our civil and moral welfare.

c. Are perhaps the most important rights granted to citizens by government in constitutions and bills of right. Movements to dilute or "balance away" these rights in the interest of national security have almost always been misdirected. Suppression of speech and movement should be carried out   only in the most extreme circumstances.

d. Are a part of the democratic heritage in the United States, but freedom doesn't mean license to say anything one wants to say at any time. There   must be strong checks on pornography

or revolutionary speech and
action.

    e. Are a myth because the corporate, capitalistic power structure through employment of the mass media conspires to suppress free and creative speech and thought.

    f. Have been grossly misinterpreted by past Supreme Court judgments. All obscene and subversive materials and actions must be suppressed to protect our country from the radical revolutionary threat at home and the planned world take-over elsewhere.

Question #8 ECONOMICS & BUSINESS.

Please read the following statement carefully. Then seek to categorize yourself roughly in one of the ways indicated.

One of the first concerns of a federal government in North America should be the provision of a sound business climate. This can be accomplished best if the government employs only minimum restrictions on businesses and corporations. For example, wage and hour legislation is basically wrong. Any contract that is developed--if there must be one--should be arranged strictly between employers and employees.

Concurrently, every effort should be made to stay with a balanced budget. In fact, an economy won't really be (safe and) sound until steady, sensible fiscal policies bring about a significant reduction in a national debt. Yet it is important, also, not to increase the burden on taxpayers even though a strong national defense is absolutely necessary. Big business is now being taxed so heavily that people's dividends on their investments are becoming unreasonably small. Inflation must be kept at a reasonable level, and the economy needs ever-present stimulation.

Through reasonable policies in re spending both at home and abroad, we should be able to develop a type of revenue-sharing in the years ahead. Through the stimulation of private enterprise, with occasional block grants of money with no strings attached made to states or provinces that are hard pressed financially, we should be able to improve the economy with a minimum of revenue-sharing that is ultimately debilitating to struggling state/provincial and local political units. We must strive always to keep people's money closer to the source from which it is produced in the first place. A federal government simply can't be "all things to all people." It is time that many of the required responsibilities and duties be returned to the state/province along with the necessary tax money to carry these tasks forward to successful conclusion.

a.   I AGREE with at this difficult time just about all of the ideas expressed in this statement.

b.   I DISAGREE generally with this statement, To me the tone seems negative. I feel that the federal government should become more involved in the control of business and industry.

c,   I DISAGREE with the statement. Laissez faire capitalism certainly helped this country initially to become strong materially. Now, however, we need somewhat more of a social-welfare state approach to meet the urgent needs of a significant percentage of the people.

d.   I AGREE GENERALLY with this statement. It seems quite sensible and reasonable. It offers positive recommendations to alleviate some of the ongoing problems that we face.

e.   I DISAGREE STRONGLY. Much of this statement is reactionary drivel. Some of these ideas may have made some sense back in the 19th century. However, the super-rich and the rich have "gotten away with murder" in North America. We simply have to figure out a way to redistribute the wealth to a reasonable extent. Democratic socialism is the answer.

f.   I AGREE STRONGLY. The labor movement and extended welfare programs have had a lot to do with the sad fiscal plight of both the United States and Canada. Budgets must be balanced, and they never will be with so many inadequate and lazy people living off the fat of the land on, for example, huge governmental payrolls. People simply must prepare themselves adequately and be willing to work. Maybe being hungry will make them look a little harder for any gainful employment.

Question #9 LAW AND ORDER.

Law and order is:

a. Clearly necessary to maintain an organized healthy society. The lack of respect for authority has led to many unfortunate incidents at all levels of society. The Supreme Court in the United States, for example, went too far in interpreting the constitutional rights of criminals. Canada has done the same thing. Maybe now we'll gradually firm up our defenses against the rising tide of people who have no fear of punishments that are typically meted out to them.

b. Now the emotional slogan of many of those individuals and groups who oppose progressive social change. Law and order without justice is characteristic of totalitarian societies. There should be no wire tapping at   all, for example. Although rioting can't be condoned, it is essential that we attack the causes of such insurrection--not the symptoms of unrest that might be inherent in our present society.

c. Essential if the free countries of the world are to survive this very difficult period. For a variety of reasons, legislatures and "supreme courts" have gone too far in coddling the truly dangerous criminal offenders without regard to public safety. In some cases jurisdictions have even gone so far as to pay criminals where they have hidden bodies of their victims.

d. The hypocritical slogan of a frightened and decadent society. The poor and minority groups occasionally strike back at the absolute, but often concealed, viciousness of an exploitive social order. "Law-'n order" tends to mean "keep Blacks, Spanish-speaking minorities, youth, and immigrants in their place!" We must treat all alike in our society.

e. The backbone of a free society. Absolutely no gains should be allowed as a result of rioting and looting with protests that get out of hand. Civil disturbances must be suppressed ruthlessly. Too many "handcuffs" have been placed on members of law-enforcement agencies doing their jobs. Maybe once again will all be able to walk the streets without fear of molestation.

f. Necessary in a democratic society, but the words as used by many take on an unpleasant overtone. Crimes rates of several types are really very serious. but we must move positively rather than negatively to reach the underlying causes and correct them. Prison rehabilitation programs must be improved significantly. I believe that crime rates would go down markedly if competency-based education and more jobs were made available.

Question #10 POPULATION CONTROL.

Please read the following paragraph. Then indicate the strength of your agreement or disagreement with the import of the statement.

The population control is starkly grim today. The situation has become now become so tragic because there are more than six billion people on earth--and the projection figure is nine billion before a declining trend is expected. We are told that all-out cooperative efforts by the major powers in the world simply cannot ward off the massive starvation of peoples that is coming in the years ahead.

Even if nutrition of an adequate nature were somehow to be provided, overpopulation is also causing staggering problems with water and stream pollution, air pollution, overcrowding in cities, etc. These difficulties will steadily great worse. A crisis of this magnitude must obviously be attacked on all fronts by people of good will worldwide.

The right to abortion should be legalized universally and readily available when there is no desire to carry a fetus through to birth. The sole choice in this matter should rest with the prospective parents (the mother in the final analysis)) with advice from a physician when requested.

Coeducational sex education should be carried out in the public schools at the earliest appropriate age. Contraceptive advice , devices when requested, should be readily available and kept at an inexpensive level with governmental subsidy if required. Subsequently, in overpopulated countries, it will probably be necessary to offer positive incentives--or even penalties!--so that the size of families will be curtailed.

Finally, we can't make the point too strongly that this vital matter has a direct relationship to world peace. There is absolutely no time to waste in the implementation of the necessary procedures to carry out the underlying philosophy expressed in the above statements.

a. AGREEMENT--The underlying rationality of this statement and the specific steps to be taken represent my position. Action is needed as soon as possible.

b. DISAGREEMENT--This is a highly personal matter. The government should refrain from direct involvement. The problem may be serious in a relatively small number of countries, but they should be able to solve it with intelligent planning.

c. STRONG AGREEMENT--This position and the implementation of the accompanying recommendations represent just a beginning. All sorts of additional measures will be needed in the future. For example, why shouldn't we have licensing so that only genetically qualified people will   be allowed to bring children into the world?

d. STRONG DISAGREEMENT--this statement is ridiculous! It goes on at length   about something that really isn't a problem. If   God had meant for people to be numbered as to the number of offspring they may produce. it   would have been so. Government has absolutely no right to become involved in such an aspect of a woman's life (or that of her mate). This whole trend should be resisted very strongly.

e. AGREE GENERALLY--population control is certainly one of the world's problems. We should work to improve the situation at home and also encourage other nations to do the same.

f. DISAGREE GENERALLY--Many have expressed concern about this problem, but it really is not as serious as they have indicated. Birth control information should be available on a voluntary basis to those whose religious faith permits such a practice.

Question #11 TRADE UNIONS.

Identify the extent of your agreement or disagreement with the following statement:

The origin, growth, and development of trade unions in North America has been most significant. When the capitalistic system reached a stage where large individual fortunes were being made, certain segments of the working population were finding it next to impossible to realize the material benefits necessary to maintain a reasonable and secure standard of living.

The advances made by unions did not come easily. In fact, the struggle was exceedingly difficult. Often long, bitter strikes were needed before reasonable--not always equitable--settlements were effected. These periodic strikes brought great hardships to many families. The concept of a "closed shop" was a bitter pill for many companies and industries to swallow. It still is for many today. The establishment of a relationship between salary raises and the cost-of-living index did not come easily either. Most helpful to the development of unions was their informal yet strong tie-ins with political parties.

The union movement has spread in many directions. This development has been very helpful to such groups as government workers, teachers. and many other occupations. Union leaders and rank-and-file members should now make strong efforts to recruit members of minority groups, women, and any other needy people at all levels of the business and commercial enterprise. This must be done, even if it becomes necessary to change existing standards temporarily--or perhaps brought about by setting up a larger number of categories. If a capitalistic economy is to exist worldwide, unions must loom large in the struggle for equality of opportunity here and everywhere else.

Unions should continue with the vigorous prosecution of their demands for such benefits as the guaranteed annual wage and other rewards to enable workers to steadily improve their quality of life. The government should not invoke the idea of compulsory arbitration except in most extreme situations to settle long-standing disputes, nor should it subject unions to back-to-work legislation except when a national emergency exists.

a. AGREEMENT--This is basically my position. The union movement gives me hope that the world is a fair place in which to live. Unions have given workers a sense of security and morale that permits them to work more productively and comfortably at the same time/

b. GENERAL DISAGREEMENT--There are some good points here, but this statement gives unions far to much credit and power.

c. STRONG DISAGREEMENT--This is ridiculous. The power of the unions must   be curbed before the overall economy is destroyed.

d. GENERAL AGREEMENT--The unions have helped North American companies, but some of these statements go too far. No group should be allowed to become too powerful.

e. DISAGREEMENT--This is definitely not my belief about the background and present position of trade unions. This development needs to be watched carefully.

f. STRONG AGREEMENT--This statement is good, but the report of accomplishments should be even more glowing. The United States and Canada would not be where they are today if it were not for the magnificent saga of North America's trade unions.

Question #12 HIGHLY COMPETITIVE SPORT.

Please record the extent to which you or disagree with the following statement:

Competitive sport was created by people thousands of years ago (presumably) to serve humankind beneficially. It can and does serve a multitude of purposes in today's world. With sound leadership it can good for both boys and girls in their formative years. It can help to develop desirable character and personality traits and also promote vigorous health. It can also provide good role models for young people to emulate. Our states and provinces should get fully behind these activities by providing appropriate competition for young people as they are developing. Such sporting competition should be regarded as supplemental to regular physical activity education programs at all levels of education.

To compete in highly competitive sport today, and do well, it requires extensive, dedicated practice over a period of many years. It is argued that it is important for our countries to be well represented in international competitions and at the Olympic Games. Thus, we should continue to find ways that we can more fully subsidize our young people so that they mat strive for, and perhaps ultimately achieve, their highest aspirations in this regard. Eventually a small percentage of these athletes will, in addition to the intrinsic rewards that sport participation provides, will search for ways to capitalize extrinsically, also on any such talent developed. In certain sports particularly enjoyed by society, these young people may even turn professional as such status becomes available to them.

Such a development takes place in a number of other life activities (e.g., music, drama), but in sport in the past this was somehow contrary to the amateur ideal and the spirit of Olympism. However, holding true to the original Olympic ideal has just about become an impossibility today. When the United States, for example, lost the Olympic title in basketball, there evidently could be only one response--bring in the "pros" with

46

their multimillion salaries to trounce those "upstarts." Now even they're having trouble "bringing home the bacon!"

As the Olympic Movement becomes increasingly professionalized at all levels, along with the problem of controlling drug usage to enhance performance, one wonders to what extent present-day practices can be compared to the problems that arose with the ancient Olympic Games. They were abolished in 776 B.C. because of the excesses that developed. We must search harder for ways to hold this cheating and phony "professionalism" in check? The question arises: Will the modern Games suffer the same fate as those of ancient times for similar reasons?

a. AGREEMENT--This is a very good statement. Sport can indeed be a force for good in the world, but we must be very careful to ensure that the evil present in many of the prevailing practices that have developed with highly commercialized sport doesn't outweigh any good that might be achieved. We are dangerously close to this now wherever the emphasis is on money largely and not on what is happening to the young man or woman involved. Many of these influences have "trickled down" to certain universities and some schools at the lower levels. We need fine programs of intramural sports for young people in all school.

b. DISAGREEMENT--This statement has some merit, but I don't buy this "good and evil" bit as described immediately above. Competitive sport has proved itself to be an important social influence in society. We need as many "winners" as possible in today's world. It's a "hard" world out there, and people need to know how to compete. Also, it is vital for our country to do well in international competition including the involvement with the Olympic Games. Further, young people who can earn athletic scholarships for their university education deserve this chance. Additionally, highly competitive sport provides a great deal of entertainment and enjoyment to millions of people as well.

Question #13 GAY AND LESBIAN RELATIONSHIPS.

47

Please read the following statement, and then decide which of the two positions is closest to your personal beliefs:

Morality and ethics have been hot topics from the 1990s on into the new century. *The New York Times* reported, for example, that "our morality is disintegrating because its foundation is eroding." The Washington Post asserted that "the core of U.S. national character has been damaged because we've lost our sense of virtue!" Although denying a person's right to choose abortion is still being argued by a minority, the question of gays in the military has been only temporarily (quite unsatisfactorily) resolved in the U.S.A.. Also, we are still finding difficulty in granting full rights as citizens to same-sex alliances. Of course, it does seem reasonable that, if a person is willing to die for his or her country in military service, how this person fulfills sexual desires in the privacy of a bedroom should hardly be a major issue today. Nevertheless, the questions of immorality and its relationship to the legal system are still with us and won't go away easily.

John Kekes, a U.S. philosopher, calls the argument that "the world is going to Hell in a hand basket," morally speaking, The Disintegration Thesis. The position is as follows:

(1) the value system of the culture no longer offers significant rationale for subordinating one's self to the common good;
(2) a healthy democratic government depends on values that come from religion (the Judeo-Christian tradition, that is);
(3) human rights are based on the moral worth that a loving God has granted to each human soul; and
(4) authority in social affairs is empowered because of underlying transcendent moral law (Brookings Institution).

What this all adds up to is that the Disintegration Thesis holds since society's basic problem is moral. What rebuttal may be offered to the idea that our culture is sliding down a slippery slope to moral bankruptcy? Kekes argues that the whole problem is simply this: Moral change has been confused with moral disintegration. He agrees that are many seemingly disturbing moral issues today, but he then inquires about the significance of these facts as a "new morality" struggles to be born. Basically what is being abandoned is the idea that there is one and only one set of virtues for a human life--One Summum Bonum, to place the dilemma in terms of Latin.

However, the Disintegration Thesis argument is that a gradual change in our morality has been occurring, and that such change will continue on into the future. However, in this change from a single morality to a pluralistic one in North America, there are still many good traits or virtues present in our daily lives. We still have the basic concepts of freedom, knowledge, happiness, justice, love, order, privacy, wisdom, etc. with which to guide and develop our personal lives and social living. However, we should understand that in this ever-increasing pluralistic culture none of these concepts is necessarily reducible to the other--and especially not to the idea that there is one transcendental moral law. This means that each person should work in his or her life for some reasonable or acceptable combination of such values as love, freedom, justice, etc.

a. AGREEMENT. I find myself essentially in agreement with the position taken immediately above by the writer. Times are indeed changing, and we simply must be fair to all concerned. A number of the concerns expressed about gay and lesbian relationships are not central to "the good life"--they are peripheral. What is important in life is that we should be fair, decent, and just in our relationships with others--not that we should concern ourselves with people's sexual preferences. A spectrum seems to exist in regard to the "maleness" or "femaleness" of a person, a condition that is inherent in that individual and cannot be altered without maladjustment occurring.

b. DISAGREEMENT. This "NEW" morality sounds great and may be all well and good to those individuals ready to accept the changes that are occurring toward a pluralistic morality. However, as a defender of The Disintegration Thesis, this argument for acceptance of such an oddly emerging situation simply adds fuel to the fire. Any individually selected amalgam of values and virtues represents just one more symptom of the moral bankruptcy that is taking place right before our eyes. The advocates of a new, more pluralistic morality, if they hope to win their argument, must show that there is sufficient continuity between the old and the new, between monistic and pluralistic morality.

Question #14 ENVIRONMENTAL CRISIS.

Please read the following statement. Then decide which of the two statements below is closest to your stance or belief about the problem outlined.

Ecology is defined as the field of study that treats the relationships and interactions of human beings and other living organisms with each other and with their natural environment. Since 1975 interest in this vital subject has increased steadily and markedly with each passing year. Nevertheless, the "say-do" gap in relation to truly doing something about Earth's plight in this regard is enormous.

What, then, is the extent of the environmental crisis in modern society? Very simply, we have achieved a certain mastery over the world because of our scientific and technological achievement. We are at the top of the food chain because of our mastery of much of Earth's flora and fauna. However, because of the explosion of the human population, increasingly greater pressures "will be placed on our lands to provide shelter, food, recreation, and waste disposal areas. This will cause a greater pollution of the atmosphere, the rivers, the lakes, the land, and the oceans" (Mergen). This bleak picture could be expanded; yet, perhaps the tide will soon turn. Certainly the gravity of prevailing patterns of human conduct is recognized by many, but a great many more people must develop attitudes that will lead them to take positive action in the immediate future. It is time for concerted global action, and we can only hope that it is not too late to reverse the effects of a most grave situation.

We can all appreciate the difficulty of moving from a scientific "is" to an ethical "ought" in the realm of human affairs. There are obviously many scientific findings within the environmental sciences that should be made available to people of all ages. Simply making the facts available, of course, will not be any guarantee that strong and positive attitudes will develop on the subject. It is a well-established fact, however, that the passing of legislation in difficult and sensitive areas must take place through responsible political leadership, and that attitude changes often follow behind, albeit at what may seem to be a snail's pace.

The field of education should play a vital role now, as it has never done before, in the development of what might be called an "ecological awareness." Obviously this has become much broader than it was earlier because the field of ecology now places all of the individual entities of Earth in a total context in which the interrelationship of all parts must be thoroughly understood. If the field of education has a strong obligation to present the various issues revolving about the newly understood need for the development of an ecological awareness, this duty obviously includes all who are employed within the educational system, have a certain general education responsibility to all participants in their classes or programs.

Presumably this matter cannot be called a persistent problem historically. The overwhelming magnitude of poor ecological practices has simply not been even partially understood by the general populace. Now some realize the urgency of the matter, but others are telling them that further study is needed, that the ecologists are exaggerating, and that they are simply pessimistic by nature.

a. AGREEMENT. I find myself in essential agreement with the underlying position taken by the writer above. This is a crisis situation because the need for "ecological awareness" is racing headlong into a collision with growing worldwide capitalism in the burgeoning global economy. The time is now to take drastic steps to alleviate and/or resolve this overwhelmingly difficult problem.

b. DISAGREEMENT. The writer makes some good points, of course. We must be ever vigilant in regard to elements and forces (also companies and people) who are careless and/or dishonest in their "relations" with the environment. However, if a country seeks to do conscientiously what it can to alleviate problems that develop, that should do the trick. The earth is resilient. This is one of a number of important and issues the world is facing.

Question #15 CLONING AND CELLULAR RESEARCH

Please read the statement below. Then record your agreement or disagreement as you did with previous questions.

In the 21st century, using a Biblical-quoting rationale based on Genesis (IV), to castigate scientists for "staggering arrogance" in presuming to play God by conducting cloning research doesn't cut much ice. (Note that god is spelled with a capital "G.") As the argument proceeds, the strength of this argument is bolstered by none other than the eminent philosopher/theologian, George W. Bush. Does the author actually think that this former Yale "scholar" personally wrote--and indeed meant!--the words he spoke? "As we seek what is possible, we must also ask what is right--and we must not forget that even the most noble ends do not justify any means"?

In response, here's a thought for our nay saying friends to absorb early in this new millennium. Your Christian God has got a tough struggle ahead to keep its status as the number #1 life force in a multiethnic world. The world society is just too replete with its many versions of "The Great One." This is becoming ever more true as both Europeans and North Americans struggle with their own rapidly increasing, multiethnic cultural incursions. Each has its "unique" version of the Almighty.

When it comes to this question of cellular and cloning research, the voices of the clerics involved come through as a "vast pooling of ignorance." They speak as though they KNOW what's right and what's wrong. They know, you see, because God told them so! The fact of the matter is that neither they--nor do any of the rest of us as their often gullible listeners--really know what's right and what's wrong anymore. Their hoary dogma simply doesn't "do it" today.

Unless knowledge of "how it all began" somehow becomes known to humankind--and can we really believe this will ever happen?--we earthlings don't have much choice. We must figure out--working together!--what's "right" action and what's "wrong" action for us in the 21st century. Our decisions quite simply must be BASED ON OUR OWN LIFE EXPERIENCE. If we don't manage to do this, ultimate disaster to life as we know it today seems almost inevitable. The handwriting is on the wall!

Cross-cultural understanding must be cultivated with great diligence. This is vital because our "global village" with its blanketing communications network is steadily bringing about similar values and norms of conduct worldwide. The world needs to view solutions to ethical dilemmas such as cloning and cellular research in a similar manner. Such an approach to ethical decision-making could well be the only hope for human life to continue successfully on Earth in the future.

a. AGREEMENT. Findings from the scientific community keep flooding in. Some are good, some debatable, and some turn out to be wrong. Life moves on in often strange and mysterious ways. It appears to be an open-ended universe. We don't really know where we came from, nor where we are going. Scientific discoveries and the medical profession backed by the health sciences have lengthened the average length of human life. Now we are promised even better length and longevity through cellular research. I say "Go for it!"

b. DISAGREEMENT. How far should humans go in tampering with life processes? When a man and woman are married and subsequently procreate. they are in tune with the plan that the Creator has preordained for humans and all other living creatures on earth. Humans should not tamper unduly with His plan for us. Abortion, for example, is a sin against humankind. Using cloned creatures for "spare parts" when or where needed is not my idea of how humans should behave.

What Was Your Score?

A. Check your answers with the following score sheet. With each question write in the appropriate number of points scored (*as plus or minus)* where indicated.

Question				Question		
1.	a.	+3		6.	a.	-2
	b.	+2			b.	+2
	c.	+1			c.	-1
	d.	-1	_____		d.	+1 _____
	e.	-2	score		e.	+3 score
	f.	-3			f.	-3

2.	a.	+3		7.	a.	+2
	b.	+1			b.	-1
	c.	-2			c.	-2
	d.	+2	_____		d.	+1 _____
	e.	-1	score		e.	-3 score
	f.	-3			f.	+3

3.	a.	-3		8.	a.	+2
	b.	-2			b.	-1
	c.	-1			c.	-2
	d.	+1	_____		d.	+1 _____
	e.	+2	score		e.	-3 score
	f.	+3			f.	+3

4.	a.	-3		9.	a.	+1
	b.	+3			b.	-1
	c.	-2			c.	+2
	d.	+1	_____		d.	-3 _____
	e.	+2	score		e.	+3 score
	f.	-1			f.	-2

5.	a.	+3		10.	a.	-2
	b.	-2			b.	+2
	c.	+1	_____		c.	-3
	d.	-3	score		d.	-1 _____

	e.	+2			e.	+1	score
	f.	-1			f.	+3	

11. a. -2   14. a. -3
    b. +1   b. +3 _____
    c. +3   score
    d. -1 _____
    e. +2 score
    f. -3

12. a. +3   15. a. -3
    b. -3   b. +3 _____
    c. -2   score
    d. +1 _____
    e. -1 score
    f. +2

13. a. -3
    b. +3 _____
            score

B. Add your plus (+) scores together (if any)..........Total = _____

C. Add your minus (-) scores together (if any).......Total = _____

D. Subtract the smaller score (plus or minus) from the larger one.

   It may be, of course, that you will have just one cumulative
   plus or minus score. In this case no subtraction is necessary.

   Your resultant total could conceivable be zero (0).
   It is more likely, however, that it will either be plus
   "something" (e,g, plus [+] 9) or minus "something" (e.g.,
   minus (-) 14.

E. The result is your Socio-Political Quotient (either conservative
   + SPQ or liberal - SPQ.

   This is not a good or bad score--whatever it is!)

Discussion

Your score could range from plus 45 to minus 45. There is a world of difference between these two extremes. The scale below is a rough approximation indicating the range of socio-political "positions." Six such positions have been identified for the purposes of this self-evaluation questionnaire.

It has been argued that a country needs both socio-political conservatives *and* liberals. Progressives are anxious to see implemented what they regard as beneficial, while conservatives want to make certain that such change being recommended is desirable and possibly beneficial *before* they accept it.

A score somewhere around the zero (0) mark is difficult to assess. It probably indicates someone who is a middle-of-the-road person, perhaps a fence-sitter on controversial issues. However, it might indicate someone who has varying positions on both sides of the spectrum--and whose scores simply balance each other out. This would be the position of an eclectic, but not what has been termed a patterned eclectic.

+33 to +45   =   (Reactionary)

+20 to +32 =   (Conservative)

+7 to +19   =   (Moderate Conservative)

+6 to -6   =   **Middle of the Road (Eclectic)**

-7 to -19   =   **Moderate Liberal**

-20 to -32   =   (Liberal)

-33 to -45   =   (Radical)

PART 3: SELF-EVALUATION

Because of my earlier background in the history and philosophy of education, and subsequent early involvement in professional preparation in my own field, I soon realized that young people thinking about entering the profession of physical activity education (and educational sport)–or whatever name the department or curriculum was designated as at some point– typically needed to undertake some serious self-evaluation. They had a lot of ideas about life, religion, education, sport and their tentatively chosen profession. However, what those ideas and thoughts added up was "another story." So I decided to develop a self-evaluation checklist to help them "get their life bearings" (so to speak). Here below in what I used with students with whom I worked. It had nothing to do with "grades in a course," of course.

WHAT DO I BELIEVE?
(A self-evaluation checklist)

> Note: I need to alert you to the fact that this "self-evaluation" is a highly subjective matter. I first developed this "personal examination" approximately 50 years ago and have updated it periodically since to the best of my ability.

Instructions

Read the statements below carefully, section by section, and indicate by an (X) *the statement in each section that seems closest to your personal belief.*

Check your answers only after all SIX sections have been completed. Then complete the summarizing tally on the answer page. Take note of apparent inconsistencies in your overall position. Finally, check with the freedom-constraint spectrum at the end to discover your educational and philosophic "location," whether in the center, the right or the left.

> Note: Many of the words, terms, phrases, etc. have been obtained from the work of philosophers, educational philosophers, recreation philosophers, and sport and physical education philosophers, living or deceased. I am most grateful

for this assistance, but finally decided *not* to mention their names individually throughout this test so as not to possibly prejudice the person taking the test. Their names are listed individually at the end, but as a group of names. In this self-evaluation check list, the *professional* sections were delimited to the professions of recreation and physical activity education (including sport).

Keep in mind that I am not seeking to make the case that, for example, a position taken under Category 1 will result *by logical deduction* in a comparable position being taken in a following category either within the education, recreation education, or physical education & educational sport categories. Nevertheless, positions taken in these latter categories should, to be consistent, probably be grounded on philosophical presuppositions stated earlier.

Category I
THE NATURE OF REALITY (METAPHYSICS)

A. _____ Experience and nature constitute both the form and the content of the entire universe. There is no such thing as a pre-established order of affairs in the world. Reality is evolving, and humanity appears to be a most important manifestation of the natural process. The impact of cultural forces upon people is fundamental, and every effort should be made to understand them as we strive to build the best type of a group-centered culture. In other words, the structure of cultural reality should be our foremost concern. Cultural determinants have shaped human history, and a crucial stage has now been reached in the development of life on the planet. Our efforts must now be focused on the building of a world culture.

B. _____ I believe that the metaphysical and normative types of philosophizing have lost their basis for justification in the 21st century. Their presumed wisdom has not been able to withstand the rigor of careful analysis. Sound theory is available to humankind through the application of scientific method to problem-solving. Thus, what is the exact nature of philosophy? Who is in a position to answer the ultimate questions about the nature of reality? The scientist is, of course, and the philosopher must become the servant of science through conceptual analysis and the rational reconstruction of language. Accordingly, the philosopher must resign himself or herself to dealing with important, but lesser, questions than the origin of the universe and the nature of the human being--and what implications this might have for everyday conduct.

C. _____ The world of men and women is a human one, and it is from the contest of this human world that all the abstractions of science ultimately derive their meaning. There is the world of material objects, of course, that extends in mathematical space with only quantitative and measurable properties, but we humans are first and foremost "concrete involvements" within the world. Existence precedes essence, and it is up to men and women to decide their fate. This presumably makes the human different from all other creatures on Earth. It appears true that people can actually transform life's present condition, and thus the future may well stand open to these unusual beings.

D. _____ Nature is an emergent evolution, and the human's frame of reality is limited to nature as it functions. The world is characterized by activity and change. Rational man and woman have developed through organic evolution over millions of years, and the world is yet incomplete. It is a reality that is constantly undergoing change because of a theory of emergent novelty that appears to be operating within the universe. People do enjoy true freedom of will. This freedom is achieved through continuous and developmental learning from experience.

E. _____ Mind as experienced by all people is basic and real. The entire universe is mind, essentially. The human is more than just a body; people possess souls, and such possession makes them of a higher order than all other creatures on Earth. The order of the world is due to the manifestation in space and time of an eternal and spiritual reality. The individual is simply part of the whole. It is therefore a person's duty to learn as much about the Absolute as possible. Within this position there is divided opinion regarding the problem of monism or pluralism (one force or more than one force at work). The individual person has freedom to determine which way he or she will go in life. The individual can relate to the moral law in the universe, or he or she can turn against it.

F. ____ The world exists in itself, apart from our desires and knowledge. There is only one reality--that which we perceive is it. The universe is made up of real substantial entities, existing in themselves and ordered to one another by extra-mental relations. Some feel there is one basic unity present, while others holding this position believe in a non-unified cosmos with two or more substances or processes at work. Things don't just happen; they happen because many interrelated forces make them occur in a particular way. People live within this world of cause and effect. They simply cannot make things happen independent of it.

Category II
ETHICS AND MORALITY (Axiology/Values)

A. ____ The source of all human experience lies in the regularities of the universe. Things don't just happen; they happen because many interrelated forces make them occur in a particular way. Humans in this environment are confronted by one reality only-- that which we perceive is it! The "life of reason" is extremely important, a position that emanates originally from Aristotle who placed intellectual virtues above moral virtues in his hierarchy. Many holding this stance believe that all elements of nature, including people, are inextricably linked in an endless chain of causes and effects. Thus, they accept a sort of ethical determinism--i.e., what people are morally is determined by response patterns imprinted in their being by both heredity and environment. A large number in the world carry this fundamental position still further by adding a theological component; for them the highest good is ultimate union with God, the Creator, who is responsible for teleological and supernatural reality. Human goodness is reached by the spirituality of the form attained as the individual achieves emancipation from the material (or the corporeal). The belief is that a person's being contains potential energy that may be guided or directed toward God or away from Him; thus, what the individual does in the final analysis determines whether such action will be regarded as right or wrong.

B. ____ There should be no distinction between moral goods and natural goods. There has long been a facts/values dualism in existence, and this should be eradicated as soon as possible by the use of scientific method applied to ethical situations. Thus, we should employ reflective thinking to obtain the ideas that will function as tentative solutions for the solving of life's concrete problems. Those ideas can serve as hypotheses to be tested in life. If the ideas work in solving problematic situations, they become true. In this way we have empirical verification of hypotheses tending to bring theory and practice into a closer union. When we achieve agreement in factual belief, agreement in attitudes should soon follow. In this way science can ultimately bring about complete agreement on factual belief or knowledge about human behavior. Thus there will be a continuous adaptation of values to the culture's changing needs that will in turn bring about the directed reconstruction of all social institutions.

C. ____ The problems of ethics should be resolved quite differently than they have throughout most of history. Ethics cannot be resolved completely through the application of scientific method, although an ethical dispute must be on a factual level-- i.e., factual statements must be distinguished from value statements. Ethics should be normative in the sense that we have moral standards. However, this is a difficult task because the term "good" appears to be indefinable. The terms used to define or explain ethical standards or norms should be analyzed logically in a careful manner. Social scientists should be enlisted to help in the determination of the validity of factual statements, as well as in the analysis of conflicting attitudes as progress is determined. Ethical dilemmas in modern life can be resolved through the combined efforts of the philosophical moralist and the scientist. The resultant beliefs may in time change people's attitudes. Basically, the task is to establish a hierarchy of reasons with a moral basis.

D. ____ Good and bad and rightness and wrongness, are relative and vary according to the situation or culture involved (i.e., the needs of a situation are there and then in that society or culture). Each ethical decision is highly individual, initially at least, since every situation has its particularity. The free, authentic individual decides to accept responsibility when he or she responds to a human situation and seeks to answer the need of an animal, person, or group. How does the "witness react to the world?" Guidance in the making of an ethical decision may come either from "outside," from intuition, from one's conscience, from reason, from empirical investigation, etc. Thus it can be argued that there are no absolutely valid ethical principles or universal laws.

E. ____ Ethics and morality are based on cosmic laws, and we are good if we figure out how to share actively in them. If we have problems of moral conduct, we have merely to turn to the Lord's commandments for solutions to all moral problems. Yet there is nothing deterministic here, because the individual himself or herself has an active role to play in determining which ethical actions will bring him or her into closer unity with the supreme Self. However, God is both the source and the goal of the values for which we strive in our everyday lives. In this approach the presence of evil in the world is recognized as a real human experience to be met and conquered. The additional emphasis here is on logical argument to counter the ever-present threat of the philosophy of science. This is countered by the argument that there is unassailable moral law inherent in the universe that presents people with obligations to duty (e.g., honesty is a good that is universal).

F. ____ Our social environment is inextricably related to the many struggles of peoples for improvement of the quality of life--how to place more good in our lives than bad, so to speak. We are opposed to any theory that delineates values as absolute and separates them from everyday striving within a social milieu. Actually, the truth of values can be determined by established principles of evidence. In an effort to achieve worldwide consensus on any and all values, our stated positions on issues and controversial matters must necessarily be criticized in public forums. Cultural realities that affect values should be reoriented through the achievement of agreed-upon purposes (i.e., through social consensus and social-self-realization on a worldwide basis). The goal, then, is to move toward a comprehensive pattern of values that provides both flexibility and variety. This should be accompanied by sufficient freedom to allow the individual to achieve individual and social values in his or her life. However, we must not forget that the majority does rule in evolving democracies, and at times wrong decisions are made. Keeping in mind that the concept of democracy will prevail only to the extent that "enlightened" decisions are made, we must guarantee the ever-present role of the critical minority as it seeks to alter any consensus established. A myth or utopian vision should guide our efforts as we strive toward the achievement of truly human ethical values in the life experiences of all our citizens.

Category III
EDUCATIONAL AIMS AND OBJECTIVES

A. _____ Socialization of the child has become equally as important as his or her intellectual development as a key educational aim. There should be concern, however, because many educational philosophers seem to assume the position that children are to be fashioned so that they will conform to a prior notion of what they should be. Even the progressivists seem to have failed in their effort to help the learner "posture himself or herself." If it does become possible to get general agreement on a set of fundamental dispositions to be formed, should the criterion employed for such evaluation be a public one, rather than personal and private? Education should seek to "awaken awareness" in the learner-- awareness of the person as a single subjectivity in the world. Increased emphasis is needed on the arts and social sciences, and the student should freely and creatively choose his or her own pattern of education.

B. _____ Social-self-realization is the supreme value in education. The realization of this ideal is most important for the individual in the social setting--a world culture. Positive ideals should be molded toward the evolving democratic ideal by a general education that is group-centered and in which the majority determines the acceptable goals. However, once that majority opinion is determined, all are obligated to conform until such majority opinion can be reversed (the doctrine of "defensible partiality"). Nevertheless, education by means of "hidden coercion" is to be scrupulously avoided. Learning itself is explained by the organismic principle of functional psychology. Acquired social intelligence teaches people to control and direct their urges as they concur with or attempt to modify cultural purposes.

C. ____ The concept of education has become much more complex than was ever realized. Because of the various meanings of the term "education," talking about educational aims and objectives is almost a hopeless task unless a myriad of qualifications is used for clarification. The term "education" has now become what is called a "family-resemblance" one in philosophy. Thus we need to qualify our meaning to explain to the listener whether we mean (1) the subjectmatter; (2) the activity of education carried on by teachers; (3) the process of being educated (or learning) that is occurring; (4) the result, actual or intended, or #2 and #3 taking place through the employment of that which comprises #1 above; (5) the discipline, or field of inquiry and investigation; and (6) the profession whose members are involved professionally with all of the aspects of education described above. With this understanding, it is then possible to make some determination about which specific objectives the profession of education should strive for as it moves in the direction of the achievement of long-range aims.

D. ____ The general aim of education is more education. Education in the broadest sense can be nothing else than the changes made in human beings by their experience. Participation by students in the formation of aims and objectives is absolutely essential to generate the all-important desired interest required for the finest educational process to occur. Social efficiency (i.e., societal socialization) can well be considered the general aim of education. Pupil growth is a paramount goal. This means that the individual is placed at the center of the educational experience.2

E. ____ A philosophy holding that the aim of education is the acquisition of verified knowledge of the environment. Such education involves recognition of the value of content as well as of the activities involved and takes into account the external determinants of human behavior. Education is the acquisition of the art of the utilization of knowledge. The primary task of education is to transmit knowledge, knowledge without which civilization could not continue to flourish. Whatever people have discovered to be true because it conforms to reality should be handed down to future generations as the social or cultural tradition. (Some holding this philosophy believe that the good life emanates from cooperation with God's grace, and further believe that the development of the Christian virtues is obviously of greater worth than learning or anything else.)

F. ____ Through education, the developing organism becomes what it latently is. All education may be said to have a religious significance, the meaning of which is that there is a "moral imperative" on education. As the person's mind strives to realize itself, there is the possibility of the Absolute within the individual mind. Education should aid the child to adjust to the basic realities (the spiritual ideals of truth, beauty, and goodness) that the history of the race has furnished us. The basic values of human living are health, character, social justice, skill, art, love, knowledge, philosophy, and religion.

Category IV
THE EDUCATIVE PROCESS (Epistemology)

A. ____ Understanding the nature of knowledge will clarify the nature of reality. Nature is the medium by which the Absolute communicates to us. Basically, knowledge comes only from the mind, a mind which must offer and receive ideas. Mind and matter are qualitatively different. A finite mind emanates through heredity from another finite mind. Thought is the standard by which all else in the world is judged. An individual attains truth for himself or herself by examining the wisdom of the past through his or her mind. Reality, viewed in this way, is a system of logic and order that has been established by the Universal Mind. Experimental testing helps to determine what the truth really is.

B. ____ The child experiences an "awareness of being" in his/her subjective life about the time of puberty--and is never the same thereafter. The young person truly becomes aware of his or her existence, and the fact that there is now a responsibility for one's own conduct. After this point in life, education must be an "act of discovery" to be truly effective. Somehow the teacher should help the young person to become involved personally with his or her education, and also with the world situation in which such an education is taking place. Objective or subjective knowledge should be personally selected and appropriated by the youth unto himself or herself, or else it will be relatively meaningless in that particular life. Thus it matters not whether logic, scientific evidence, sense perception, intuition, or revelation is claimed as the basis of knowledge acquisition, no learning will take place for that individual self until the child or young person decides that such learning is "true" for him or her. Therefore the young person knows when he or she knows!

C. ____ Knowledge is the result of a process of thought with a useful purpose. Truth is not only to be tested by its correspondence with reality, but also by its practical results. Knowledge is earned through experience and is an instrument of verification. Mind has evolved in the natural order as a more flexible means whereby people adapt themselves to the world, Learning takes place when interest and effort unite to produce the desired result. A psychological order of learning (problem-solving as explained through scientific method) is ultimately more useful than a logical arrangement (proceeding from the simple fact to the complex conclusion). However, we shouldn't forget that there is always a social context to learning, and the curriculum itself should be adapted to the particular society for which it is intended.

D. ____ Concern with the educative process should begin with an understanding of the terms that are typically employed for discussion purposes within any educational program. The basic assumption is that these terms are usually employed loosely and often improperly. For example, to be precise we should be explaining that a student is offered educational experiences in a classroom and/or laboratory setting. Through the employment of various types and techniques of instructional methodology (e.g., lectures), he or she hears facts, increases the scope of information and/or knowledge, and learns to comprehend and interpret the material (understanding). Possessing various kinds and amounts of ability or aptitude, students gradually develop competencies and a certain degree or level of skill. It is hoped that certain appreciations about the worth of the individual student's experiences will be developed, and that he or she will form certain attitudes about familial, societal, and professional life that lie ahead. Finally, societal values and norms, with other social influences, will help educators, fulfilling role within their collectivities and subcollectivities, determine the best methods (with accompanying experimentation, of course) of achieving socially acceptable educational goals.

E. ____ An organismic approach to the learning process is basic. Thought cannot be independent of certain aspects of the organism. This is because thought is related integrally with emotional and muscular functions. The person's mind enables him or her to cope with the problems of human life in a social environment within a physical world. Social intelligence is actually closely related to scientific method. Certain operational concepts, inseparable from metaphysics and axiology (beliefs about reality and values), focus on the reflective thought, problem-solving, and social consensus necessary for the gradual transformation of the culture.

F. ____ There are two major learning (epistemological) theories of knowledge in this philosophical stance. One states that the aim of knowledge is to bring into awareness the object as it really is. The other emphasizes that objects are "represented" in the human's consciousness, not "presented." Students should develop habits and skills involved with acquiring knowledge, with using knowledge practically to meet life's problems, and with realizing the enjoyment that life offers. A second variation of learning theory (epistemological belief) here indicates that the child develops his or her intellect by employing reason to learn a subject. The principal educational aims proceeding hand in hand with learning theory here would be the same for all people at all times in all places. Others with a more religious orientation holding this position, basically add to this stance that education is the process by which people seek to link themselves ultimate with their Creator.

Category V
VALUES IN RECREATION (EDUCATION)

A. _____ As I see it, work and play are typically sharply differentiated in life. Play serves a most useful purpose at recess or after school, but it should not be part of the regular curriculum. I believe that the use of leisure is significant to the development of our culture, but I realize today that improved educational achievement is going to take a lot more hard work and somewhat less leisure. I see leisure pursuits as an opportunity to get relief from work while serving a re-creative purpose in human life. So does the more recent bio-social theory of play--the idea that play helps the organism to achieve balance. I feel that the "play attitude" is missing almost completely in most competitive sports. Play (and recreation) are, therefore, very important to me; I believe they should be "liberating" to the individual. People can develop their potentialities for wholesome hobbies through recreation. Further, recreation can serve as a "safety valve" by the reduction of the psychic tensions that are evidently caused by so many of life's typical stresses. In sum, even though play should *not* be considered as a basic part of the curriculum, we should not forget that it provides an "indispensable seasoning" to the good life. Along with a sound general education, *extra-curricular* play and recreational activities should suffice to equip the student for leisure activities in our society.

B. _____ I believe that all types of recreational needs and interests should be met through recreation education. The individual should have an opportunity to choose from among social, aesthetic and creative, communicative, "learning," and physical recreational activities within the offerings of what might be called a "community school" in the broadest sense of the word. It is absolutely imperative, of course, that these choices be made according with the student's desire to relate to people. All students are striving for self-realization, and the recreation education program can promise opportunities for both individual expression, as well as for group recreational undertakings. Play seems necessary for people of all ages, and it can assume many different forms. We should not forget that one of its functions is simply personal liberation and release.

C. _____ I believe it is difficult to separate the objectives of recreation education from physical education when physical activities are being considered. Within the schools I recommend a unified approach for health, physical education, recreation education, and dance. In this discussion I am only including those recreational activities that are "physical" in nature. All these leisure activities should be available to all students on a year-round basis. I see recreation education as a legitimate phase of the core curriculum, but later in the day I would include additional recreational opportunities as well as opportunity for relaxation. In a core curriculum so-called extracurricular activities are quite as integral as "spoke and hub" activities. In fact, the word "extra" has now become most misleading.

D. _____ I am inclined to adopt the adoption of the name recreation education for the field. I see advantages in a unified approach whereby the four specialized areas of health, physical education, recreation, and dance (in schools) would provide a variety of experiences that would enable the young person to live a richer, fuller life through superior adjustment to the environment. I believe that education for the worthy use of leisure is basic to the curriculum of the school, a curriculum in which pupil growth, as defined broadly, is all-important. Secondly, play should be conducted in such a way that desirable moral growth will be fostered. Thirdly, over-organized sport competition is not true recreation, since the welfare of the individual is often submerged to the extreme emphasis that is so frequently placed on winning. I believe it is a mistake to confuse the psychological distinction between work and play with the traditional economic distinction generally recognized. All citizens should have ample opportunity to use their free time in a creative and fruitful manner. I do not condemn a person who watches others perform with a high level of skill in any of our cultural recreational activities, including sport, so long as the individual keeps such viewing in a balanced role in personal living.

E. _____ I believe that the role of play and recreation in the development of personality and the "perfectly integrated" individual is looming larger with each passing year, and that such a role has not been fully understood or appreciated in the past. For this reason it seems quite logical to me that education should re-assess the contributions that recreation and play do make in the overall education of the student. That there is a need for further educational research along these lines is self-evident to me. I believe further that we should examine very closely any theories of play and recreation that grant educational possibilities to these activities of people. The self-expression theory of play, for example, suggests that the human's chief need in life is to achieve the satisfaction and accomplishment of self-expression of one's own personality. Here is an explanation that considers quite fully the conception of the human as an organic unity, a total organism. I believe that a person is a purposive being who is striving to achieve those values that are embedded in reality itself. To the extent that we can realize the eternal values through the choice of the right kinds of play and recreation without flouting the moral order in the world, we should be "progressive" enough to disregard a dualistic theory of work and play. Another difficulty that confronts us is differentiating between physical education and recreation. Recreation in its totality has developed to the point where it is now clearly one of our major social institutions. I believe that recreation can make a contribution to the development of an "integrated individual in an integrated society growing in the image of the integrated universe." Humankind today, as I see it, is faced with a "recreational imperative."

F. _____ I believe that there is a radical, logically fundamental difference between statements of what is the case and statements of what ought to be the case. When people express their beliefs about recreation education, their disagreements can be resolved in principle. However, it is logical also that there can be sharing of beliefs (facts, knowledge) with radical disagreement in attitudes. In a democracy, for example, we can conceivably agree on the fact that people of all ages should be involved in wholesome recreational activities of all types, but we can't force people to get actively involved or even to hold a favorable attitude toward such activity. We can demonstrate tenable theory about such recreational involvement, but we cannot prove that a certain attitude toward such activity is the correct one. Thus I can accept evidence that specific types of recreational activity may bring about certain effects or changes in the individual, but my own attitude toward subsequent regular involvement--the values in it for me--is the result of a commitment rather than a prediction.

Category VI
VALUES IN PHYSICAL ACTIVITY EDUCATION
(including EDUCATIONAL SPORT)

A. _____ I believe in the concept of total fitness which implies an educational design directed toward the individual's self-realization as a social being. In education, for example, there should be an opportunity for selection of a wide variety of useful human motor performance activities relating to sport, exercise, dance, and play is necessary to provide a sufficient amount of "physical" fitness activity. The introduction of dance, music, and art into physical education can contribute to the person's creative expression. Intramural sports and voluntary physical recreational activities should be stressed. This applies especially to team competitions with particular stress on cooperation and the promotion of friendly competition. Extramural sport competition should be introduced when there is a need. Striving for excellence is important, but it is vital that materialistic influences should be kept out of the educational program. In today's increasingly stressful environment, relaxation techniques should have a place too, as should the concept of education for leisure.

B. _____ I believe that the field of physical activity education & educational sport should strive to fulfill a role in the general education pattern of the arts and sciences. The goal is total fitness, not only physical fitness, with a balance between activities emphasizing competition and cooperation. The concepts of universal man and universal woman are paramount, but we must allow the individual to choose his or her sport, exercise, and dance activities for himself or herself based on knowledge of self and what knowledge and/or skills he or she would like to possess. We should help the child who is "authentically eccentric" feel at home in the physical education program. It is also important that we find ways for youth to commit themselves to values and people. A person should be able, and be permitted) to select developmental physical activity according to the values he or she wishes to derive from it. This is often difficult in our society today because of the extreme overemphasis placed on winning--being Number 1! Finally, creative movement activities such as modern dance should be stressed, also.

C. ____ I believe that education "of the physical" should have primary emphasis in the field of physical activity education. I am concerned with the development of physical vigor, and such development should have priority over the recreational aspects of sport and physical education. Many people who hold the same educational philosophy as I do recommend that all students in public schools should have a daily period designed to strengthen their muscles and develop their bodily coordination and circulo-respiratory endurance. Sport and physical activity education must, of course, yield precedence to intellectual education. I give qualified approval to interscholastic, intercollegiate, and interuniversity athletics, since they help with the learning of sportsmanship and desirable social conduct if properly carried out. However, all these objectives, with the possible exception of physical training, are definitely extracurricular and are not part of what we call the regular educational curriculum.

D. ____ I am much more interested in promoting the concept of total fitness rather than physical fitness alone. I believe that sport and physical education should be considered an integral subject in the curriculum. Students should have the opportunity to select a wide variety of useful activities, many of which should help to develop "social intelligence." The activities offered should bring what are considered natural impulses into play. To me, developmental physical activity classes and intramural-recreational sports are much more important to the large majority of students than highly competitive athletics offered at considerable expense for the few. Thus physical education and sport for the "normal" or "special" young man or woman deserves priority if conflicts arise over budgetary allotment, staff availability, and facility use. However, I can still give full support to "educational" competitive sport, because such individual, dual, and/or team activities can provide vital educational experiences for young people if properly conducted.

E. _____ I believe that there is a radical, logically fundamental difference between statements of what is the case and statements of what ought to be the case. When people express their beliefs about physical education and (educational) sport, their disagreements can be resolved in principle. However, it is logical also that there can be sharing of beliefs (facts, knowledge) with radical disagreement in attitudes. In a democracy, for example, we can conceivably agree on the fact that jogging (or bicycling, swimming, walking, etc.) brings about certain circulo-respiratory changes, but we can't force people to get actively involved or even to hold a favorable attitude toward such activity. We can demonstrate tenable theory about the benefit of such physical involvement, therefore, but we cannot prove that a certain attitude toward such activity is the correct one. Thus I may accept evidence that vigorous sport, dance, exercise, and play can bring about certain effects or changes in the organism, but my own attitude toward subsequent regular involvement--the values in it for me--are the result of a commitment rather than a prediction.

F. _____ I am extremely interested in individual personality development. I believe in education "of the physical," and yet I believe in education "through the (*medium* of the) physical" as well. Accordingly, I see physical activity education (including sport) as important, but also occupying a lower rung on the educational ladder. I believe that desirable objectives for physical education and sport would include the development of responsible citizenship and group participation. In competitive sport, I believe that the transfer of training theory is in operation in connection with the development of desirable personality traits (or undesirable traits if the leadership is poor). Participation in highly competitive sport should *always* serve as a means to a desirable end (often a dubious premise in today's overly emphasized competition).

> Note: Appreciation should be expressed at this point to the following people from whose work phrases and very short quotations were taken for inclusion in the checklist. Inclusion of their names at those particular points in the text did not seem

advisable, inasmuch as the particular position or stance may have been instantly recognized: John S. Brubacher, Abraham Kaplan, Morton White, William Barrett, E.A. Burtt, Van Cleve Morris, Ralph Harper, Herbert Spencer, J. Donald Butler, George R. Geiger, Theodore Brameld, John Wild, Harry S. Broudy, James Feibleman, Roy W. Sellars, Isaac L. Kandel, Alfred N. Whitehead, Mortimer J. Adler, Wm. McGucken, Pope Pius XII, Herman H. Horne, Theodore M. Greene, Wm. E. Hocking, and Paul Weiss.

Answers

Read only after the question under each of the six categories have been completed. Record your answer to each part of the checklist on the summarizing tally form below.

I. The Nature of Reality (Metaphysics)

   a. Strongly Progressive (Reconstructionism, Brameld)
   b. Analytic (a philosophic method, not a stance))
   c. Existentialistic (atheistic, agnostic, or theistic)
   d. Progressive (Pragmatic Naturalism; Ethical Naturalism)
   e. Traditional (Philosophic Realism, with elements of Naturalistic Realism, Rational Humanism, and positions within Catholic educational philosophy)--Type "B"
   f. Traditional (Philosophic Idealism)--Type "A"

II. Ethics (Axiology)

   a. Traditional / Type "B"
   b. Progressive
   c. Analytic
   d. Existentialistic
   e. Traditional / Type "A"
   f. Somewhat Progressive

III. Educational Aims and Objectives

a. Existentialistic
b. Somewhat Progressive
c. Analytic
d. Progressive
e. Traditional / Type "B"
f. Traditional / Type "A"

IV. The Educative Process (Epistemology)

a. Traditional / Type "A"
b. Existentialistic
c. Progressive
d. Analytic
e. Somewhat Progressive
f. Traditional / Type "B"

V. Recreation

a. Traditional / Type "B"
b. Existentialism
c. Somewhat Progressive
d. Progressive
e. Traditional / Type "A"
f. Analytic

VI. Physical Education & Educational Sport

a. Somewhat Progressive
b. Existentialistic
c. Traditional / Type "B:
d. Progressive
e. Analytic
f. Traditional / Type "A"

Table 1
Summarizing Tally For Self-Evaluation

Category   I
Metaphysics

_____

Category   II
Ethics &
Morality

_____

Category   III
Educational

Objectives

_____

Category   IV
Epistemology

_____

Category   V
Recreation

_____

Category   VI
Physical Activity
Education (including
Educational Sport)

_____

Totals					
P	SP	EX	AN	TR (A)	TR (B)

Further Instructions

It should now be possible--keeping in mind the subjectivity of an instrument such as this--to determine your position approximately based on the answers that you have given and tallied on the form immediately above.

At the very least you should be able to tell if you are progressive, traditional, existentialistic, or analytic in your philosophic approach (or stance).

If you discover considerable eclecticism in your overall position or stance--that is, checks that place you on opposite sides of the freedom-constraint spectrum, or some vacillation with checks in the existentialistic or analytic categories--you may wish to analyze your positions or stances more closely to see if your overall position is philosophically defensible.

Keep in mind that your choices under Category I (Metaphysics or Nature of Reality) and Category II (Axiology/Values) are basic and==in all probability--have a strong influence on your subsequent selections.

Now please examine the freedom-constraint spectrum below. Keep in mind that "Existentialistic" is not considered a position or stance as the others are (e.g., Traditional or Philosophic Idealism). Also, if you tend to be "Analytic," this means that your preoccupation is with analysis as opposed to any philosophic/theologic system-building.

Finally, then, after tallying the answers (your "score" above), and keeping in mind that the goal is not to pigeonhole you forever, did this self-evaluation checklist show you to be:

( ) Strongly Progressive--FIVE or SIX checks left of center on the spectrum?

( ) Progressive--FOUR or FIVE checks left of center?

( ) Somewhat Progressive--FOUR checks left of center?

( ) Eclectic--Checks in two or three (?) positions on both the right and left of the spectrum's center?

( ) Somewhat Traditional--FOUR checks right of center?

( ) Traditional--FOUR or FIVE checks right of center?

( ) Strongly Traditional--FIVE or SIX checks right of center?

( ) Existentialistic--FOUR or FIVE checks (including Category I) relating to this stance?

( ) Analytic--FOUR or FIVE checks (including Category I) relating to this approach to doing philosophy?

Figure 3

The Freedom-Constraint Spectrum

Eclectic*

Existentialistic**
(atheistic, agnostic,
or theistic)

Traditional
(Idealism)

Somewhat Progressive
(Reconstructionism;
Brameld)

Traditional
(Naturalistic Realism,
including Communism)

Progressive
(Pragmatic Naturalism)

Traditional
(Rational Humanism)

Strongly Progressive
(Naive Naturalism)

Strongly Traditional
(Scholastic Realism)

ANARCHY
"the left"

DICTATORSHIP
"the right"

Analytic Orientation--a philosophic outlook, actually with ancient origins (as opposed to metaphysical or normative philosophizing), that moved ahead strongly in the twentieth century. The assumption has been that our ordinary language has many defects that need correction. There is concern also with conceptual analysis. Another objective is "the rational reconstruction of the language of science" (Abraham Kaplan). The basic preoccupation is with analysis as opposed to philosophical system-building based on metaphysical and/or normative methodology.

* So-called *eclecticism* is placed in the center because it assumes that the person evaluating himself or herself has selected several positions or stances on opposite sides of the spectrum. Most would argue that eclecticism is philosophically indefensible, while some believe that "patterned eclecticism" (or "reasoned incoherence" as a few have called this position) represents a stance that many of us hold.

** *Existentialistic-Phenomenological Orientation*--a permeating influence rather than a full-blown philosophical position; there are those with either an atheistic, agnostic, or theistic orientation. This position is shown slightly to the left of center because within this "tendency" there is a strong emphasis on individual freedom of choice.

PART 4
GUIDING STUDENTS TO LITERACY
IN PHYSICAL ACTIVITY EDUCATION

"There was a field called physical education.
With so many names it writhed in frustration.
Still it dithered and blathered while peregrinating,
and finally died silently while still ruminating."

It would be neither wise nor kind at this time to criticize--or perhaps even make a bit of fun of, as was done immediately above in the note--earlier leaders in the field of physical (activity) education for the present plight the field faces. In fact it would be very difficult to say precisely where and when the field "went wrong" during the twentieth century. For example, was there a critical incident at which point the die was cast? Suffice it to say that there are now well over 200 different, multi-faceted titles presumably describing what is intended to be the subject-matter composition of these present-day educational units--professional and/or disciplinary--at the college and university levels in the United States of America.

In addition to what has happened with programs for physical and health education in the schools, of course, we now also have some 300-400 professional curricula in sport management, as well as a "multitude" of programs where the term "kinesiology" in prominent. In both cases the end goal is different with sport management being a professional curriculum and kinesiology designated as a disciplinary one where the science of movement is stress throughout.

Although the development of the concept of "the allied professions" began early in the 20th century, a critical incident in the development of the field of physical education as a so-called profession-but really a subject matter within education-was the decision of the American Academy of Physical Education (AAPE) to change its name to the American Academy of Kinesiology and Physical Education (AAKPE). A full explanation of the reasons behind this change will not be presented here. Subsequently--with the guidance of Editor Janet C. Harris of *Quest* and Karl M.

Newell's argument that use of the term *kinesiology* would help to bring "chaos out of order--the entire issue of *Quest* (Vol. 42, No. 3, December, 1990) was devoted to a discussion of this development by various theorists in the field. In that issue Daryl Siedentop stated (pp. 320-321) "Newell and I disagree fundamentally on the nature of the field. I believe it to be a professional field. I believe persons who want to serve in the field need to be prepared in a professional program. . . ." To this author the intent of Siedentop's statement is crucial to the future development of a profession that should be called *physical activity education.* What follows here is an effort to explain how those who now still call themselves "physical educators" at heart and in practice might recover from this present plight. The question is asked whether they can ever fulfill what was intended to be their original mission, thereby becoming vital to the provision of healthful, developmental physical activity for the country's population.

This halcyon state could possibly be achieved if those responsible for professional preparation in ??? guided *qualified* professional students to full literacy in a discipline increasingly being called *kinesiology* while at the same time (or subsequently) preparing them *professionally* in *physical activity education.* If this were to become the norm, and these graduates were imbued with a life purpose to provide people of all ages and conditions with purposeful, developmental physical activity, physical activity educators could create a nation of healthy, vigorous people that would set an example for the world.

This does appear to be the way things are going in North America. Increasingly students are completing a *disciplinary* curriculum titled kinesiology that precedes (or in some cases coincides) successful completion of a series of classroom and laboratory course experience that also qualify the student to receive a *professional* teaching certificate from the state or province in which the courses were taken.

Then, completely separate from kinesiology, there is the development labeled "sport management" where some 300-400 colleges and universities now sponsor a degree program with that title with courses leading to a bachelor's degree. And, at the graduate level, we now find a master's degree and a doctorate in sport management as well. Obviously the basic undergraduate program in sport management would be, and is, significantly different from that of kinesiology as well as that of-say-physical & health education. (This will be explained further below.)

Definitions

1. The meaning used for the term "literacy" here is *the second one* provided in the *ENCARTA World English Dictionary*, 1999, p. 1052)--i.e., "knowledge of, or training in, a particular subject or area of activity." (The first definition given is "the ability to read and write to a competent level.") Further, the meaning of the term in this analysis has been broadened to mean *professional* literacy--*i.e., the expert knowledge and competencies held by the professional practitioner.*

2. The term *"kinesiology"* is defined as the discipline or body of knowledge about human movement in exercise, sport, and physical recreation
.

3. The term *"physical activity education"* is defined as the knowledge, competencies, and skills relating to exercise, sport, and physical recreation that can be taught to children and young people in educational institutions, as well as to adults of all ages throughout their lives in various situations and environments.

4. The term *"physical activity educator"* is defined as that person who uses the knowledge and competency available about developmental physical activity to teach a planned program of physical activity education either in the educational system or in society at large.

5. The term *"sport management"* is defined as the knowledge, competencies, and skills relating to the management of sport and related physical activity for people of all ages.

6. *Managerial achievement* at a given time results from the execution of managerial acts by a person with excellent personal skills, involving further conceptual, technical, human, and

conjoined skills, while combining varying degrees of planning, organizing, staffing, directing, and controlling within the management process to assist an organization to achieve its stated goals.

Cultural Literacy

The reader may wonder why the terms "literacy" and now "cultural literacy" are being introduced into this discussion. The reason is that clarification of the full meaning of the terms is needed. Actually, part of the problem that the field of physical education has faced is that many people feel that its professional practitioners themselves often have not achieved full literacy-- literacy based on the *first* definition of the term in a dictionary (see "Definitions" immediately above). Whether physical activity educators are good readers and writers--as all professional people should be--is not the primary concern of this discussion at the moment, however. What is needed now is to explain that the "literacy" needed for *professional practitioners* is provided in the second definition provided above under "Definitions"--i.e., the expert knowledge *and competency* desired for the physical activity educator. Such "literacy" would be "professional literacy" that is over and above the "cultural literacy" recommended for all Americans by Prof. E. D. Hirsch in the late 1980's (1988, 1991).

Before discussing expert knowledge and professional competency further, however, it is important to clarify the subject of cultural literacy somewhat further. Hirsch believes that it is their common knowledge or collective memory that "allows people to communicate, to work together, and to live together," and that "if it is shared by enough people, it is a distinguishing characteristic of a national culture," "one that makes each national culture unique" (p. ix). After publishing *Cultural literacy*, a book in which he explained his conception of it, he took the next logical step, with associates Joseph Kett and James Trefil, to publish *The dictionary of American literacy* in 1988. The "cultural knowledge" included in this unique volume was stated to be what every literate American of the late 20th century ought to know, or at least be familiar with if not known fully and precisely. Such cultural knowledge is simply that mass of information that is to be preserved along with any additional information meeting the definition that is constantly being added to the "mass" as time passes.

If this "cultural literacy" is "the foundation of our public discourse," and it is "what makes Americans American," then the authors had to establish certain rules that would apply to this assemblage of information. First, they decided not to include specialized information that would be known only by experts, while at the same time leaving out basic information that was "below" what they termed necessary cultural literacy. Second, they decided to include only that information or item that would presumably be known by a majority of *literate* Americans. Finally, they did not include current events that would not have enduring significance to the society, or at least a strong possibility of achieving such status. These exclusions and inclusions, they felt, would give cultural literacy a "lasting significance" (p. x). Interestingly, and disturbingly, the authors decided that what happened in competitive sport, plus what they called "entertainment," in America was too "ephemeral" to include-- with notable exceptions (e.g., Lou Gehrig, Babe Ruth). (This decision appears to be most unfortunate because, if art, music, and dance have been included under "Fine Arts" as cultural forces--which they should be, of course--then, for better or worse, sport too has become a very strong cultural influence in America. It is now possibly even too strong a social force; so, its omission would seem to be an error in judgment, made possibly through bias.)

Hirsch and his colleagues have certainly given all of us interested in general education something to think about. When the declining statistics of such basic information are known, how can anyone argue with the proposition that "achieving high universal literacy ought to be a primary focus of educational reform in this country"? (p. xi). They argue that what they call "true functional literacy" is fundamental to a successful society because it is what "is holding the social fabric of the nation together." The authors assert also that: "true literacy depends on a knowledge of the *specific* information that is taken for granted in our public discourse." They insist that true literacy involves "acts of communication" that "requires a knowledge of shared, taken-for-granted information" that lies "below" the written page. On the surface of things, their rationale provides a strong argument for attempting to counteract the decline in what is called "national literacy" in their discussion (p. xi).

The authors explain further why there is a "high correlation between reading ability and learning ability." They stress how important is that a reader be able to comprehend various types of writing. They argue that "to have a good *general* reading ability, the student needs to know about a lot of things." Taking this argument still further, they state that "language arts are also knowledge arts." Having pointed out that "high reading ability is a multiplex skill that requires knowledge in a wide range of subjects," Hirsch et al. declare that the same thing can be said about *learning* ability. If we can associate something new with something that we learned previously, we are literally combining the new idea with similar older ideas or concepts already mastered. All of this--learning more and more about the world in which we live--adds up to the need for people to have as broad a background knowledge as possible.

It was important to explain what cultural literacy is meant to be and where it fits into the educational scheme provided for the literate citizen. Cultural literacy is general information that helps us communicate with friends, business associates, and strangers alike. However, professional literacy in what is here being called physical activity education is the main topic for consideration in this discussion. (Or it would be *sport management* for that professional field, and *kinesiology* for the discipline involving the study of human movement.)

Physical Activity Education

Throughout Part 4 the author will argue that the term *physical activity education* would be a better term for a field that wishes to turn out full-fledged professional educators--one that conceivably serves people of all ages and conditions in twenty-first century schools and communities. The following are three basic reasons for this assertion:

1. It has long been argued that the term physical education implies a tri-partite division of the human organism. Educational essentialists were said to believe in education *of* the physical dimension of a person, whereas educational progressivists countered with an "education *through* the physical" argument. The latter approach now coincides with the belief in psychology that the human organism is indivisible. Nevertheless, this quibbling between factions in the field made it very difficult for physical education to make its case in the educational hierarchy throughout the twentieth century. Unfortunately this opprobrium against physical (activity) education still exists today in some quarters both within the educational milieu and in the public domain.

2. The term "physical (activity) education" has somehow become identified with a learning experience that takes place in a gymnasium in an educational institution only. As such it has often been associated in people's minds with dull, routine-like exercises and similar uninteresting experiences that they don't want to repeat for the rest of their lives after school years are over.

3. For several years the term "physical activity" has been used by various professional and disciplinary groups instead of the term "exercise." The assumption is that people don't like being told that they *have* to exercise. For example, *Physical Activity Today* is a publication put out by the Research Consortium of the American Alliance for Health, Physical Education, Recreation, and Dance. Also, the Presidents Council on Physical Fitness and Sport has substituted the term "physical activity" for "exercise." Further, Health Canada, a governmental group, in collaboration with ALCOA (Active Living Coalition for Older Adults) and CSEP (Canadian Society for Exercise Physiology) publishes *Canada's Physical Activity Guide* and makes it available free of charge. Thus, physical activity implies a variety of activities such as walking, exercising, sports, and types of physical recreation. It now seems, therefore, that physical activity education, may well be the most desirable term to take the place of physical education.

If this proposal were accepted generally, the professional preparation program or curriculum in a university would be designed to prepare a physical activity educator as a qualified professional educator. Depending on the standards set, this person could also qualify for subsequent certification or licensing by the state or province (1) as a teacher in the public schools, (2) as a professional physical activity educator in private practice, or (3) as a professional physical activity educator in a private, semi-public, or public agency.

Such achievement would constitute a guarantee to the public and other hiring officials that the graduating professional student had completed a thoroughgoing, competency-based, physical-activity education program in which:

> (1) professional functions and needs were ascertained,
> (2) individual competencies were specified,
> (3) necessary performance levels were determined,
> (4) program content and instructional methodology were defined, and
> (5) competency attainment, as specified at the outset, was carefully evaluated.

Professional Preparation Development
for the Physical (Activity) Educator

Down through the years of the 20th century many educators urged that there should be a stronger "cultural" component in the professional curriculum of the physical education teacher. However, although some progress was made, the demands for strengthening the other curriculum areas (i.e., foundation arts and sciences, professional education requirements, health education courses) limited the extent to which this objective could be reached. A number of studies indicated also a lack of standardization in course terminology within the developing specializations of the overall field of health education, physical education, and recreation (Zeigler, 1962)

There were many attempts to improve the *quality* of professional preparation through studies, surveys, research projects, national conferences, and accreditation plans. A significant text recommending a "competency approach" to the preparation of teachers was published (Snyder and Scott, 1954). The field had been continuing to move toward ongoing self-evaluation and improvement. The American Association for Health, Physical Education, and Recreation (subsequently "the Alliance") was a great influence in this historic development. It was aided significantly by such affiliated groups as the College Physical Education Association (later the NCPEAM) and the National Association of Physical Education for College Women (NAPECW), both of which merged to form the National Association for Physical Education in Higher Education.

The American Alliance for Health, Physical Education, Recreation, and Dance has long since asserted that each of the terms in its name represents separate professions (or fields of endeavor) that are nevertheless also almost inextricably allied. Interestingly, the International Council for Health, Physical Recreation, Sport and Dance has recently added the term "sport" to its title as well. The term "physical education" has also been joined with the word "sport" for some time in the National Association for Sport and Physical Education within the Alliance, but the Alliance's name remains unchanged. Interestingly, although the Canadian Association for Health, Physical Education, Recreation and Dance has followed the lead of its counterpart in the United States.. However, physical and health education remain closely intertwined; in fact, the former CAHPERD is now PHE Canada and its publication is called *Physical and Health Education Journal*. Dance educators have also been active traditionally within PHE Canada.

What has been a most significant development in both countries is the inauguration in the 1960's of a great variety of separate sub-disciplinary and "sub-professional" societies in each country that are often conjoined as North American societies (e.g., the North American Society for Sport History). For better or worse, a large majority of the scholars trained in physical education graduate programs originally have now transferred their primary allegiance to these more broadly North American societies as well. Also, a devastating blow to the field of physical education was the fracture in the relationship between the Alliance (AAHPERD) and the former American Academy for Kinesiology and Physical Education (AAKPE), a move caused by a perceived need to separate the discipline from the profession. (The latter society is now the National Academy of Kinesiology.) However, it can be argued that it occurred also because of certain state legislators' concern about the term "education" in the school curriculum and possible personality conflicts within the Alliance and the Academy. These two organizations (AAHPERD and NAK [formerly AAKPE]) had historically met annually in a conjoint fashion to the great benefit of both groups. Meeting separately now means that upwards of 100 of kinesiology and physical activity education's finest scholars and researchers are to all intents and purposes removed from the strong *professional* milieu of the Alliance. Funds for professional travel can only be stretched so far; hence, attendance figures decline…

These developments described immediately above have taken place largely within the last half of the 20th century and the first decade of the 20th century, although some of the "subdivision" that has occurred within what was earlier known as *physical education only* started earlier (e.g., health education, recreation). *What is significant in all of these individual movements, of what may be called either a professional or "sub-disciplinary" nature (e.g., recreation or sport psychology, respectively) is that they were efforts by professional people and/or scholars and researchers to specialize in the related fields of study (i.e., the sub-disciplinary and sub-professional components of the field)..*

This movement of professionals and scholars, either within the Alliance or outside of it, has left the field of physical education in a precarious, untenable situation. Now to be a qualified physical educator in the eyes of one of more groups or jurisdictions, the prospective teacher was confronted with a number of difficult hurdles. In fact, the difficulty of overcoming these "obstacles" became apparent to this author when completing an unpublished master's degree study on the topic more than 60 years ago. He concluded that a five-year program of study was needed instead of the four typically required for state certification. It was found that it was simply impossible to guarantee (1) a broad general education, (2) a creditable major in physical education including foundation subjects, (3) an acceptable minor in a related teaching area, and (4) the requisite number of professional education courses (including student teaching) in a four-year curriculum.

A Need for Redirection and Rejuvenation

Diagnosis of the present situation indicates that the field long known as physical education throughout the 20th century needs *redirection* and *rejuvenation* as the field moves along in the new century. As difficult as it may be, the profession must come to grips with the fact right now that "physical educators" are still typically "jacks-of-all-trades and masters of none!" This is what they have been, and this is what they are presently. Can it possibly be argued that this a good thing, or is it bad and should such a casual description of the field be changed? After many years of involvement, the author has now come to believe that the field of physical (activity) education, technically speaking, is a segment of the education profession. Hence, it has a duty and responsibility to work its way through to an appropriate name and a consensual taxonomy of required knowledge and competencies for its work in the field of education. Every self-respecting profession has a body of knowledge that practitioners should (must?) master to practice effectively. What is the body of knowledge in physical (activity) education? What are the specific competencies and skills this person should possess? Where is all of this explained? (Additionally, where is the "body of knowledge" for sport management and for kinesiology, respectively? More about this soon...)

Agreement about a name for the field, a complete taxonomy for its subject matter, the steady, ongoing development of an under-girding body of knowledge, and a list of the required competencies needed could reasonably soon place the field in a position where a professional practitioner would be recognized as a "such-and-such" no matter what type of position that person held within the field--or for that matter in which state or territory such professional service was carried out. Reaching consensus will undoubtedly be "horrendously difficult." However, it is now absolutely essential that these two fields (i.e., physical [activity] education and sport management strive for such an objective. Right now one is continually forced to the conclusion that physical educators have over the decades become "jacks of all trades, masters of none." (Conversely, in a much shorter period of time, the essential aspects of the profession of sport management have been delineated clearly!) Frankly, something must be done about physical (activity) education! The time has come to bring the field's image into sharper focus for the sake of the futures of professional students, not to mention the public at large (Zeigler, 1997).

How the Field of "Physical (Activity) Education"
Should React to the Arrival of the Discipline of "Kinesiology"

Now I will discuss why the physical activity educator within the public education system, who is also concurrently concerned also with related health and safety education, should not worry basically about the fact that many colleges and universities are giving the name "kinesiology" to their related administrative units in which their first training unit is located. Lest the reader rise up in anger immediately and declare that I am a traitor to the field (i.e., physical education) in which I have labored lo these past 70 years, my only request is to hear me out: There is one caveat to what I have just said. My statement of approval holds *ONLY IF* in the process the quality of subsequent *professional* education received on the way to the baccalaureate degree remains at a high level!

To understand the ramifications of the prevailing situation where "complete confusion reigns" in North America-and probably elsewhere too-as to what the many respective units should be named is a fairly long story. To address it accurately and fairly is the purpose of this essay. Historically, human physical activity has had a simultaneously glorious and shameful existence. It is a part of the very nature of the human world. This is an incontrovertible fact. It affects both the animate and inanimate aspects of our existence. It is a basic part of the fundamental pattern of living of every creature that has ever lived on the miniscule planet called Earth.

Early men and women knew human physical activity was important, but it was often not appreciated until it was gone, or almost gone. Semi-civilized men and women used it extensively in the early societies, as did the ancient Greeks and Romans and all others since. Some used physical activity vigorously, while others used it carefully and methodically. Human physical activity was used (1) gracefully by some, (2) ecstatically by others, (3) rigorously by many when the need was urgent, and (4) regularly by the vast majority who simply wanted to get the job done or enjoy themselves thereafter. Human physical activity was called many things in various tongues. But, strangely enough, it was never fully understood in a scientific sense.

The time came when human physical activity was considered less important in life. "Physical workers" earned less than "mental" workers. Yet people still admired it when a human performed skillfully on special occasions. Some seemed to understand human physical movement instinctively, while others had great difficulty in employing it well. However, human physical activity in daily life was eventually degraded in modern society to such an extent that well-educated people often did not think that it had an important place in preparation for life. Others paid lip service to the need for it, but they, in the final analysis, would not give it its due. Others appreciated its worth in what could be termed "animal fitness," but also felt it was less important than other aspects of education.

Nevertheless, planned human physical-activity movements persisted despite the onset of an advancing technological age. Some called it calisthenics. Others called it physical training. A determined Germanic group called it gymnastics, as ancient Greeks had done earlier. A few called it physical culture, but they unfortunately were thought to be men of "ill repute." Others felt that it had been neglected in the preparation of the human for life. So, they did it a "favor" and called it "Physical Education"! (If they only knew...)

The Aftermath of a New Name

Physical education gradually prospered to a degree with this

92

name, although, for many, this term was embarrassing because it classified PE as a second-class citizen in a mind-body-spirit triumvirate. This idea persisted even though, early in the 20th century, psychologists "declared" that the human organism was "unified." This effectively killed the belief that the mind and body were separate. However, as they say, long–held beliefs die hard! Nevertheless, physical education struggled on. Then an unexpected development happened: because it gained a modicum of prosperity, organized physical education "spawned" offshoots. Two of these offshoots had been closely related to PE since the early human societies arose; they were known as dance and athletics (i.e., sport). Out of these grew two new offshoots. One became known as recreation to be enjoyed when "free time" first became available, and the other as health & safety education as humans learned more about such concepts. Our "hero" (physical education or PE) helped to develop them significantly, and they–in their gratitude-helped physical education too as they themselves became more important, even vital.

In the early years of the 20th century in America, someone knew enough Greek to apply the term "kinesiology" to a course treating the study of human movement in the professional physical education curriculum in North America. Today, 100 plus years later, that name may be the title given not only to that course, but also to myriad departments, schools, and faculties in universities across North America. Interestingly, also, in Ontario, Canada, if a person holding a degree in *physical education* (where he/she took and passed one course in kinesiology) dared to call himself/herself a kinesiologist *without holding a degree with that specific name on the proverbial sheepskin*, that person would be liable to a fine of $25,000 due to legislation enacted on behalf of the Ontario Kinesiology Association! That's what I call "progress"!

The term "kinesiology" itself is evidently from the Greek language and means "the study of movement." Although this is technically correct, the advocates of this name change a generation ago may or may not have known that the verb *kineo* was also a very common Greek verb that describes the movements of sexual intercourse. This the writer learned from Prof. Doug Gerber of Classical Studies The University of Western

Ontario, Canada at explained that in Aristophanes' comedy Lysistrata the women of Athens are portrayed as going on a "sex strike" to get their husbands to end a war that they detested. As Professor Gerber explained, there "is a long scene between a husband and wife in which the husband desperately tries to get his wife into bed, and the wife uses every trick to hold him off until he agrees to vote for peace." What was the husband's name? You guessed it. Kinesias. Interestingly, the "Kinesias war" has extended down to the present day…

Then, after two world wars and numerous smaller ones, along with the significant impact of other social forces on society in this or that post–war society, physical activity education–still a second-class citizen among educators–discovered that its offshoots (recreation and health & safety education) had grown fairly large and important in the world. They too were anxious to become first-class citizens, and they made "loud noises "on occasion to inform all that they deserved greater priority in life. Many people–at least a good portion of them– recognized that they were right. However, times change slowly, and this recognition only slightly influenced educational practices.

During this same period, two other phenomena took place that held great import for physical education. PE's brothers and sisters, athletics and dance, had been performing so well that they had steadily grown stronger and more powerful. Athletics (or "sport" as it is called on some continents other than North America) looked at "PE" and said: "What a dull clod art thou!" What did athletics (sport) mean by that? Physical activity education, or training for human physical movement, wasn't very exciting. Actually it could be quite dull, what with its repetitive muscular exercises and endurance activities that promote muscular strength, flexibility, and cardiovascular efficiency.

Sadly also, dance (PE's other "relative") seemed to feel the same way. PE realized, of course, that s/he had a responsibility to teach young people about developmental physical activity in schools, but could understood it was so much more thrilling to perform for the cognoscenti (as with dance), and even for the multitudes (as with sport). So dance said: "I'm an art. So I think

94

I'd be better served by joining my fellows in one of the performing arts centers springing up *all* around me." Then, truly troublingly, athletics (sport), although very popular both as an extra-curricular activity, and also out in the public sector commercially, "moved in "and became the major part of many PE classes...

If matters weren't bad enough, Sputnik – the first artificial satellite – was launched in 1957 and the world has not been the same since. "Science" became the watchword in the 1960s and has continued as such ever since; a development that has had a profound effect on physical education. A president of Harvard University, in a report, sharply criticized professional preparation for physical education as being "shallow". This resulted in a discovery among many university professors that they no longer wanted to be known as *"physical* educators". They seemed a little ashamed to be called "that", believing that it hurt their chance to increase status, which in turn reduced the availability of much-desired grant funding. So, instead, the name "kinesiology" was proposed in various quarters.

Then, too, in the 1980s, some state legislators in the United States challenged the quality of courses that included the word "education" in their titles. And–you guessed it!-physical *education* got caught up in the melee. In addition, the American Academy of Physical Education added the term "Kinesiology" up front in its overall title. This move was to be a panacea for beleaguered academics ("if they don't know what it is, how can they criticize it?"). This lead to an assumption that goes: "granting agencies will be more apt to open up their coffers because they don't know what it is!" so it must be new and "more scientific".

> Note: Since then, not only has the term 'physical education' been dropped from the official title, the Academy is now called the National Academy of Kinesiology! Additionally, the assumption about granting agencies seems to have been true as well...

Interestingly, this study-of-movement name (Kinesiology), a word taken from the Greek language, had been the name of a course in the professional physical education curriculum for over a century. It could be "fathomed" quite well *kinematically* by most folks, but not *kinetically* by 99% of us. Now it was also to become *the* name for the department or school in a university where courses related to human physical movement were offered. Advocates were saying: "Let 'PE' be for the name for elementary and secondary school classes; kinesiology should be the "in name" for us scientists in the universities!" (Question: What then was to become of the social-scientists and humanities scholars in our field?) Still another faction, mostly in Canada, seized upon the term "kinetics" and put the word "human" before it. This sounded good too, but it is identical with both the prevailing name for dynamics in the field of physics and of that for studying rates of reaction within the field of chemistry. This led some to ask: Why should we muddy the waters further?

The effort to "scientize" 'PE' – a trend that began in the 1960s – gradually became a solid thrust designed to promote defensible *theory* to underlie practice in the realm of physical education and athletics administration. This soon got caught up and slowed by both "scientification" and budgetary restrictions in the 1970s. When this movement returned in the 1980s with enhanced budgets, however, the die had been cast even though many academic departments struggled along with unique and disparate nomenclature that has extended to the present. Also, unfortunately the overemphasis on commercialized sport both within education and in the public sector continued. As concerned professors in NCAA Division I and II were wont to say: "We don't have any problem with what's going on in athletics; they're 'over there'!"

The Unhappy Plight of Physical Education:
"Good Old 'PE'"

All of this "ancient history" made (PE) physical (activity) education become more worried than ever before. Human movement could look back at a long heritage going back to the time in the development of the universe when creatures from the sea moved onto the land mass. In addition, PE could rationalize that people with pure motives simply misjudged the importance of human physical activity. People have always seemed to treat physical educators as less bright than teachers of other subjects, even though deep down they admired physical skill. In addition, they knew that they themselves needed regular physical activity involvement themselves. Nevertheless, when seemingly intelligent people with lesser physical skill themselves discussed PE, their lips tended to curl even though they might themselves be fat (or obese!), or diabetic, or – dare I say it – lazy...

Hence, thinking about the proverbial rose, fringe physical educators increasingly wondered if they would "smell as badly" with another name. Another name was recommended, a new, concocted disciplinary name such as "phyactology" (Fraleigh). Such a name made sense in the absence of a satisfactory name, but "savants" laughed when it was first proposed... Time for reconsideration?

Time for Reflection

Finally PE began to think deeply – that is, as deeply as a second-class citizen with limited intelligence can think. PE's male proponent had a "twin sister". This female creature often made different noises as she went her own way during the second half of the twentieth century. She had been telling "the male PE" person that he couldn't see the forest for the trees. "PE," she said, "we have really been fools, and we merit our plight. We have been so stupid that we haven't been able to spell out what we really should have been called. We are involved with human physical activity or *movement*. This would probably not be a good name for an academic department, but developmental physical activity might do well as disciplinary nomenclature for a departmental title in higher education. But by all means let's make it a term that people can understand!

Human physical movement can be understood when scientists and scholars realize that here is a name that is simple to pronounce, and people can understand it superficially at least. Perhaps the field's true function can be understood more purposely than ever before using the term *developmental physical activity*. People can be helped to realize that there is more to "movement" than push-ups and jogging, as truly important as these physical activities might be. They can understand, also, that the field has physiological aspects, anatomical aspects, psychological aspects, philosophical aspects, sociological aspects, historical aspects – and many more than could be counted on the fingers of two hands.

However, even though this was a most important realization for *physical activity educators* who, annually, are being more fully under girded by a sound scientific and scholarly basis, the time was still not ripe for acceptance Even though the field's name might then be spelled correctly and the case for recognition might be soundly based, and the field could be defined as "the interaction of the human and his/her movements" (Paddick). Or, if you will, broaden it to Kenyon's term: "human movement arts and sciences." Or the "arts and sciences of human physical activity."

Good old "PE" suddenly felt very tired. Should s/he change names again? "Kinesiology" sounds so complicated and esoteric. What we are fundamentally, s/he thought, is human physical activity in sport, dance, play, and exercise. Our knowledge base comes from what might be called the movement arts and sciences or developmental physical activity, a field that can help humans throughout their entire lives.

Those who would do good in this world cannot expect others to roll stones out of their path. It's a hard road that lies ahead. But if this road is to be traversed, it must be done by a determined, united group of qualified, professional physical activity educators under girded by a solid scholarly foundation. If this means that the "academic" or "disciplinary" name under girding our field within universities will be called "kinesiology," *so be it*!

How "PHE" Should React to "Kin"…

If that were the end of the story, and "everyone lived happily ever after", that would be a wonderful result. Regardless of the introduction of a "foreign name," the terminology employed does correctly translate as "the study of movement." However, we are finding today that kinesiology has also become a convenient "umbrella" for a growing variety of professional and possibly disciplinary-oriented people who believe that it is the ideal term for them to use as they working assiduously to see to it that it is presumably used correctly by the people truly entitled to use it for their purposes. One of this group of kinesiologists could well be the director or coordinator of a physical activity and health education program that includes intramural sport competition that is included as a required subject in the school curriculum from kindergarten on up through Grade 12 of the secondary school curriculum. Such a person would begin as a student by matriculating in, and graduating from, a four-year university program in a recognized educational unit that was entitled to put the word "kinesiology" on his/her diploma upon graduating. Presumably, then, over and above such disciplinary training, the person involved then would have to have pass a sufficient amount of theory and practice courses that would qualify him/her to be granted a teaching certificate in the North American state or province in which such professional service as a teacher would occur.

Most of these "kinesiologists" today have as their goal the provision of professional service to humankind through the medium of human movement. They are typically qualifying themselves professionally–based on the information stated in their website–to serve in areas of professional practice as a certified kinesiologist or in one instance as a researcher in the discipline of kinesiology) as follows:

> Clinical Kinesiologist
> Ergonomist
> Rehabilitation Coordinator
> Private Consultant
> Clinic Manager
> Work Site Analyst
> Researcher
> Business Owner
> Occupational Health and Safety Specialist
> Work Disability Consultant
> Vocational Rehabilitation Specialist
> and many others…

Note: The term "researcher" implies that *only the person* in this category had qualified as a graduate of a program granting a disciplinary degree... All of the other terms used relate to either a profession or a trade. Interestingly, the term "professional educator in physical and health education", does not appear in this listing, although only

Further, in the words of the Ontario Kinesiology Association:

Certified Kinesiologists assess human movement, performance, and function by applying the sciences of biomechanics, anatomy, physiology, and psychomotor behavior. They work in a variety of roles and are employed in both the public and private sector. They are professionals who have obtained a university degree from a recognized university. Kinesiologists are typically involved in the rehabilitation, prevention, and management of disorders to maintain, rehabilitate, or enhance movement, function or performance in the areas of sport, recreation, work, and exercise. Kinesiologists also provide consulting services, conduct research, and develop policies related to rehabilitation, human motor performance, ergonomics, and occupational health and safety (information adapted from www.oka.ca).

At this point in this discussion of how members of the field of *physical activity and health education* within the education profession should react to what has happened to the curriculum known as physical education that began in 1861 in America. I wish it were possible to postulate: "all would live happily ever after!

Further, and this really concerns me, I believe that physical & health educators should be kinesiology graduates in the sense that they should truly understand human movement technically (i.e., both kinematically *and* kinetically) *as well as, socially and philosophically*. If this were to happen, then perhaps people who serve the field of physical & related health education within the education profession could separate themselves from should be considered as ancillary coaching duties and responsibilities. In addition, these kinesiologists serving the field of education in this way might truly understand that their mission is either to become kinesiology scholars and researchers, or to work as physical activity educators with ALL of the children in school.

Looking to the Future

As we look to the future at a time when physical activity education and related health and safety education is needed so greatly at all levels o education, I have come to believe that we should come together in the struggle that has been going on in connection with related terminology describing who we are and what it is that we do.

I well recall the communication I had in 1994 from the erstwhile dean who served the Faculty of Kinesiology at The University of Western Ontario so very well, Dr. Bert Taylor. He believes that "the name change was inevitable and necessary". He felt that "it gave us [at Western] instant credibility on campus and most certainly with the science granting agencies." As he explained further, "we were pigeons as 'PE' holed up with the concept of athletics and not regarded as a true academic discipline." Taylor argued further that "some of the exceptional young researchers we and others have been able to hire would have been lost if we were still 'PE'." Finally, Taylor stressed that we truly belong as "one strong unit" within a faculty of health sciences. Hence, the time may have well come when we must not haggle and debate the issue any longer, since the sun is already quite high in the sky... Long live *human physical activity*, because without *it* you're dead!

A Proposed Taxonomy for the Curriculum in Kinesiology & Physical Activity Education

What then should be the composition of the curriculum in kinesiology & physical activity education? In the late 1970's the author began to deplore the rift that had seemingly inevitably developed in the field since the mid-1960's between the so-called scholars and the so-called practicing professionals. The reader may remember what happened--that is, the rift between the people who were not ashamed to be called "physical educators" and those who were. As time has shown, there are now the self-proclaimed kinesiologists or "human kineticists" seeking academic respectability in our universities by calling themselves "what they ain't!" Typically they can't truly analyze human movement! Those anxious to accept the term "kinesiology" for use as the name of the former physical education unit on college and university campuses should move slowly and cautiously before changing their department's name. Somehow very few graduating physical education/kinesiologists end up being able to analyze movement kinematically, much less kinetically. And yet this is what the term "kinesiology" means literally--the study of movement! Also, as it has turned out, the offerings of various departments and schools of kinesiology differ significantly. One school of kinesiology (unnamed!) offers, for example, a variety of areas of concentration: health and physiological science, human/factors/ergonomics, active health, and biomedical engineering. Interestingly, many of these units designated as kinesiology are more than meeting their admission quotas. It is true, also, that certain people in these departments of kinesiology have been deprecating those old-fashioned units at other universities still adhering to the name "physical education." Yet do we really know what their students specializing in kinesiology do after they graduate?

Granting that "a rose by any name smells the same." The term "kinesiology" is from the Greek language and does indeed mean "the study of movement." Although this may be technically correct, the advocates of this name change in lieu of "physical education"--at the university level at least--evidently don't know (or care?) that the verb *kineo* is also a very common Greek verb that describes the movements of sexual intercourse. And the husband's name in Aristophanes' famous *Lysistrata*, the comedy where the women of Athens go on a sex strike to get their husbands to end a war--you guessed it!--was *Kinesias*. Further, to "add insult to injury," those units that have adopted the term "human kinetics" should keep in mind that kinetics is actually a subdivision of another department on campus--the department of physics!

The author recalls the words of the great C. H. McCloy, State University of Iowa, written to the author more than a half century ago. Wrote he, "The name 'physical education' is now so solidly entrenched that changing it would be akin to rolling back Niagara Falls." This feat has indeed now been accomplished on occasion. Where does that leave a field called "physical education." What does all of this add up to? Simply this: if physical education doesn't take positive steps to rectify this ongoing decline and continuing trend, it will continue to lose "professional ground."

What can possibly be done about these myriad problems? One approach would be to develop a taxonomy that would include both the professional and disciplinary dimensions of the field With this thought uppermost, it was postulated that a "balanced approach" between the *sub-disciplinary* areas of the field and what might be identified as the *sub-professional* or concurrent professional components was desirable. By this was meant that what many have called scholarly professional writing (e.g., in curriculum theory, management thought and practice) will be regarded as scholarly endeavor if done well, just as what many have considered to be scholarly, scientific endeavor (e.g., in the exercise sciences) if done well should indeed be regarded as professional writing too (i.e., writing that should ultimately serve the profession).

As part of an effort to close what was regarded as a debilitating, fractionating rift within the field, a taxonomical table was developed to explain the proposed areas of scholarly study and terms only) along with the accompanying disciplinary and professional aspects. There was agreement on eight areas of scholarly study and research that are correlated with their respective sub-disciplinary and sub-professional aspects in Table 1 above. Most importantly, the reader will note that the names selected for the eight areas *do not include terms that are currently part of the names of, or the actual names, of other recognized disciplines* and that are therefore usually identified with these other (related) disciplines primarily by colleagues and the public (Zeigler, 1982, p. vii)

Table 1
UNDERGRADUATE CURRICULUM
IN KINESIOLOGY & PHYSICAL ACTIVITY EDUCATION

Areas of Scholarly Study & Research	Sub disciplinary Aspects	Sub professional Aspects
I. BACKGROUND, MEANING & SIGNFICANCE	-History -Philosophy -International & Comparative	-International Relations -Professional Ethics
II. FUNCTIONAL EFFECTS OF PHYSICAL ACTIVITY	-Exercise Physiology -Anthropometry & Body Composition	-Fitness & Health Appraisal -Exercise Therapy
III. SOCIO-CULTURAL & BEHAVIORAL ASPECTS	-Sociology -Economics -Psychology (individ.& social) -Anthropology -Political Science	-Application of Theory to Practice
IV. MOTOR LEARNING & CONTROL	-Psycho-motor Learning -Physical Growth & Development	-Application of Theory to Practice
V. MECHANICAL & MUSC. ANALYSIS OF MOTOR SKILLS	-Biomechanics -Neuro-skeletal Musculature	-Application of Theory to Practice
VI. MANAGEMENT THEORY & PRACTICE	-Management Science Business Admin.	-Application of Theory to Practice
VII. PROGRAM DEVELOPMENT	Curriculum Studies	-Application of Theory to Prac.

(General education; professional preparation; intramural
sports and physical recreation; intercollegiate athletics;
programs for special populations--e.g., handicapped--
including both curriculum and instructional methodology)

| VIII. MEASUREMENT & EVALUATION | Theory about the Measurement Function | -Application of Theory to Prac. |

The Field Should Develop and Promote
Its Own Discipline Within The Profession of Education

The position being taken here now is that the field-since it and others accidentally or purposely have developed their own discipline-should now promote and continue to make to *create its own discipline* (i.e., kinesiology). In the process the *profession* of education should continue to have the field of physical activity education taught by physical activity educators as described above. At the same time the practitioners in physical activity education should be working cooperatively with their related disciplines and allied professions (to the extent that such cooperation is possible and useful in relation to the problems jointly faced).

There is an important point to be made at this juncture. Continuing to speak of *sociology* of sport, *physiology* of exercise, etc., is making these other disciplines and professions awaken to the importance of what physical activity educators in the past believed to be *their* educational task (i.e., the gathering and dissemination of knowledge about developmental physical activity through the media of sport, exercise, and related expressive movement–and also the promotion of it to the extent that such promulgation is socially desirable).

Such "awakening" by people in the related disciplines and allied professions is necessarily not a bad thing, of course. For example, it happened in the historical aspects of the field when it was reported in *The Chronicle of Higher Education* in the 1970's that sport history had been discovered. As a matter of fact, as of 1969 there were already 54 physical education doctoral studies and hundreds of master's theses on *purely* sport history (Adelman, 1971) Additionally, there has been literally thousands of physical education theses and dissertations with a historical orientation over the past 80 years! Further, the North American Society for Sport History has held conferences and published a scholarly journal since the early 1970's, and there was also a fine *Canadian Journal of Sport History*. This encroachment on what was considered to be its domain should cause the field of physical (activity) education no concern, however, if its primary emphasis were to shift to what is known about *developmental physical activity* and how this knowledge may be used effectively and efficiently in *physical activity education*!

The reader can certainly understand, however, that there is a different serious concern being expressed here. The end result of a continuation of this splintering of the so-called profession of physical education-that is really a field of study!-is bound to result in a "mish-mash" of isolated findings by well-intentioned, scholarly people not in a position to fully understand the larger goal toward which the field of physical (activity) education has been striving. It can be argued that the field is gradually becoming doomed to perpetual *trade* status--not *disciplinary or professional* status--composed of perennial "jacks-of-all-trades, masters of none." The field should clarify its "field status," because it is being outflanked by so many different specialists and specialties--including kinesiology (or human kinetics)--that one hardly knows in what area physical education as a self-described profession can speak authoritatively. If physical educators don't take positive steps to rectify this continuing trend in their field's development by changing their image, it will continue to lose "professional ground" while functioning with a subject-matter still considered an unimportant, expendable part of the educational curriculum.

It doesn't have to be this way. However--and this is vital! -- the situation would change dramatically if the present field of sport and physical education (NASPE's designation) were subdivided and the physical education segment were to become physical activity education (e.g., changing its title from NASPE to NAPAE). (Here it is being assumed that there would [or could] be a separate association for sport and/or sport education.) A separate *field known as physical activity education has the inherent potential to serve the high goal of enriched living and well-being for all people.* It could provide an opportunity for the improvement of the quality of life and, additionally, there is now evidence that regular exercise throughout one's life will lengthen one's lifespan as well. These are tremendously important reasons for every man, woman, and child to want to strive for an ongoing state of physical well-being. No other professions can make such a claim, but a field called physical activity education could do this best for people of all ages and conditions with the accompanying help of its allied fields (e.g., health education) and related discipline (i.e., kinesiology). Moreover, no other field will (or can) do this for what is now called physical education! However, because of physical education's inability or unwillingness, other professions and trades are arguably now fulfilling some of its duties and responsibilities--*but in a piecemeal fashion!* This can only result in sporadic, incomplete knowledge, competencies, and skills coming belatedly and ineffectively to help people improve the quality of their lifestyles.

An Inventory of Scientific Findings
About Developmental Physical Activity
Is Needed Right Now

What is needed right now, and is not presently available, is a steadily growing, categorized inventory of scientific findings about *kinesiology* in exercise, sport, physical recreation, and expressive movement arranged as *ordered generalizations* to help professional practitioners *in physical activity education* in their daily work. Physical activity education, as it is being called here, does not have this knowledge and information readily available for daily use by its practitioners. Such emerging knowledge is fundamental for the finest level of educational practice for teachers, coaches, managers, supervisors, and others engaged in positions of a public, semipublic, or private nature (e.g., YMCAs and commercial fitness establishments).

Ordered Principles or Generalizations

To make these ordered generalizations available and current, the professional association should devise and develop a series of ordered generalizations about developmental physical activity in sport, exercise, and related expressive movement and make them available to professionals both online and in the form of a loose-leaf, expandable handbook. What exactly are *ordered principles* or *generalizations?*.

Ordered principles or generalizations are simply important and verified findings about (1) what we really know, (2) what we nearly know, (3) what we think we know, and (4) what we claim to know. These principles or generalizations are arranged in an ordered, 1-2-3-4 arrangement--*and in as plain English as is possible!*

As an example, taken from the field of management theory (one of the sub-professional divisions of developmental physical activity explained in Table 1 above), the following findings about "the organization," arranged as *ordered* principles or generalizations have been extracted from Berelson & Steiner (1964, pp. 365-373):

The Organization.

A1   The larger, the more complex, and the more heterogeneous the society, the greater the number of organizations and associations that exist in it.
        A1.1   Organizations tend to call forth organizations: if people organize on one side of an issue, their opponents will organize on the other side.
        A1.2   There is a tendency for voluntary organizations to become more formal.

A2   There is always a tendency for an organization (of a non-profit character) to turn away, at least partially, from its original goals.
        A2.1   Day-to-day decisions of an organization tend to be taken as commitments and precedents, often beyond the scope for which they were initially intended, and thus affect the character of the group.
        A2.1a   The very effort to measure organizational efficiency, as well as the nature of the yardstick used, tends to determine organizational procedures.

A3   The larger the organization becomes, the more ranks of personnel there will tend to be within it.

[Etc.--keeping in mind practical limitations, of course.]

A Plan Leading Toward an Ever-Expanding Body of Knowledge Through the Implementation of a System Approach

An initial effort has been made above to present the "why" and "what" of a proposed online inventory of scientific findings covering developmental physical activity as it relates to the field, but now it is time to discuss the "how" in relation to the way in which this proposed development can be effected. It has been recommended further that such an inventory be based on a revised taxonomy including both the sub-disciplinary and the sub-professional aspects of the profession.

The first such inventory of ordered principles or generalizations would assuredly have certain gaps or deficiencies caused obviously by present inadequacy.   Such an inventory of the discipline of *developmental physical activity* or the proposed profession of *physical activity education* should be arranged primarily for *"our own"* use. The basic difference between what is presently available through several sources (e.g., SIRC) is that, in addition to bibliographic data, articles, etc., it would provide the *first* version of an ordered set of generalizations as described in the example immediately above. This version would have obviously leave much to be desired. There would be no need for apology, however, because such an effort would represent a meager beginning compared to what may be possible in 10, 20, or 50 years. However, this development will not come about unless substantive change in present practice occurs .

To this end, a recommendation is being made here for the gradual implementation of a systems approach, so that (1) university personnel relating to the discipline, (2) professional practitioners in the field, (3) scholars and researchers in other disciplines and professions, and (4) the general public could visualize the scope of the development needed to make available a sound, complete body of knowledge about developmental physical activity. This service is needed *right now* and should be made available as soon as possible in such a way that it can be called up instantaneously--either as a bibliographic listing, an abstract, a complete article, *or as a series of ordered generalizations indicating where this new knowledge coincides or clashes with present understanding.*

Along with many other fields, those scholars relating to kinesiology, as well as those teaching physical activity education do not yet appreciate the need to promote and subsequently implement a "total system" concept. There are many urgent reasons why the field must take a holistic view if the discipline and most closely related profession hope to merit increased support in the future. The promotion of this "evolving entity" of developmental physical activity, characterized as it is with so many dynamic, interacting, highly complex components, would require the cooperation of innumerable local, state or provincial, national, and international scholarly and professional associations and societies so that full support for the total professional effort could be provided.

The model presented here to help achieve a common purpose for developing and using theory and research (Figure 1) explains a system with interrelated components that could be functioning as a unit--admittedly with constraints--much more effectively than it is at present! Although in practice the execution of such an approach would be complex, the several components of the model being recommended are basically simple. As can be observed from Figure 6 below, the cycle progresses from *input to thruput to output* and then, after sound consumer reaction is obtained and possible corrective action is taken, moves back to input again (possibly with altered demand or resources) as the cycle is renewed (Zeigler, 1990, p. 218a).

Taking the first step toward the development of an inventory of scientific findings, one designed to meet the needs of North Americans primarily, would also have relevance for professional laboratory experiences from which would result the competencies and skills necessary to perform as a successful professional practitioner. (It could also be studied profitably in an ancillary manner by students wishing to specialize in either health and safety education or recreation and park administration, but it has

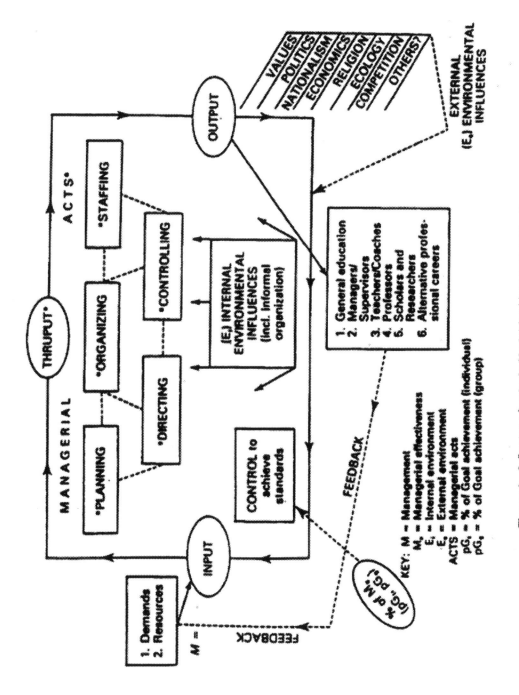

Figure 6. A System Analysis Model for Managerial Effectiveness in a Professional Preparation Program for Sport & Physical Activity Managers

KEY: M = Management
M_e = Managerial effectiveness
E_i = Internal environment
E_e = External environment
ACTS = Managerial acts
pG_i = % of Goal achievement (individual)
pG_g = % of Goal achievement (group)

111

not been designed to meet the needs as an introduction to either of these developing professions. Moreover, students intending to specialize in sport coaching or dance education as developing professions could use it to advantage as an introduction to developmental physical activity because the focus should be on human movement in exercise, sport, physical recreation, and expressive movement.)

In any analysis of this emerging field that traces the developments of the twentieth century, three categories or subdivisions of the field should be investigated:

(1) the growing and potential body of knowledge being created by researchers and scholars drawing upon research methods and techniques of the sub-disciplinary areas;

(2) the similar development of knowledge emanating from the concurrent professional components of the developing field (as exist in all subject-matter fields to a greater or lesser extent); and

(3) the knowledge becoming available from what may be called the allied professions.

Competencies and Skills Required
for Professional Literacy

It should be made crystal-clear at this point that, *in addition to mastery of the necessary knowledge base*--in a thoroughgoing competency-based approach should be employed throughout the professional program so that the competencies, and skills deemed necessary are acquired to the desirable extent. This experiential approach represents one more effort to direct professional preparation away from the stereotypical *"mastery of the textbook approach"* employed throughout the twentieth century. (In addition to making available a *broadly based* knowledge component that--through textbooks, lectures, and related literature--should be mastered prior to receiving a baccalaureate degree, such an evolving body of information should also be available on-line in the form of *ordered generalizations* for qualified, registered professionals in the field wherever they might be located.)

What follows will seek to explain how the author and his colleague (Gary Bowie) deviated from "the standard approach" in relation to one subject-matter area of the eight displayed in the model for the discipline proposed in Table 1 above--i.e., management theory and practice related to physical education and (educational) sport (Zeigler and Bowie, 1995). (It should be made clear that this same *experiential* or *laboratory* approach is being recommended for learning in *each* of the other seven categories displayed in Table 1 above (e.g., functional effects of physical activity, curriculum theory & program development) of the overall discipline designated as developmental physical activity.) The authors proceeded on the assumption that the time was past due to develop a text that truly related to management *competency* development for trainees who would later themselves be administering programs in physical activity education. What resulted was unique in that it was the first time that an "experiential" or laboratory approach had been employed throughout an *entire* administration text in the field. The result was a workbook or manual that could be used *independently* or even in conjunction with what was considered a standard text (i.e., one that had little or no *practical* exercises in it). Thus, the instructor was in a position to involve the students in "laboratory experiences" that were developed from well over 100 desirable experiences tabulated under five broad management competency categories.

The five broad competency categories for use in the experiential approach were determined after a comprehensive analysis of management science literature. From many sources the predominant thought was that there was a need to introduce a step-by-step plan for management competency or skill attainment. In doing so in connection with this investigation, a decision was made to build on Katz's (Harvard) tri-partite categorization (1974). The end result included five subdivisions in which the *personal* attributes needed for the administrator of physical activity education, as well as those *"conjoined"* skills gained through a "combinatorial" process that the individual is often required to employ on the job. What Katz called *human* skills, were now called *interpersonal* skills so as to distinguish them from personal skills (# 1 below). These subdivisions or categories of administrative skills are as follows:

1. Personal skills (or developing one's own individual competencies prior to concentrating on the managerial task).
2. Interpersonal skills (or acquiring the skills needed to influence people positively to work toward accomplishment of organizational objectives and goals).
3. Conceptual skills (or learning to formulate ideas and plans while on the job as an administrator).
4. Technical skills (or acquiring the various skills and techniques needed to cope with the various organizational details and problems that arise).
5. Conjoined skills (or developing the various managerial skills in some combination or proportion to achieve both immediate objectives and long-range goals). (Zeigler & Bowie, 1995, p. 111).

This plan enables the teacher and the students to move selectively from theory to practice within each of the five subdivisions or categories shown above. The method for working toward the achievement of the specific competencies or skills is as follows:

(1) through the provision of statements describing the objectives of the modules used to develop the competencies,
(2) to offer "knowledge statements" introducing the trainee to the theoretic bases of the competencies and their roles and functions in the management process, and
(3) by recommending selected laboratory exercises for achieving a degree of success (at least!) based on involvement in a variety of problem-solving experiences.

After the student comprehends the problem to be met or solved, a questioning process determines:

   (1) what needs to be known,
   (2) where this information may be obtained,
   (3) how to organize the actual learning experience,
   (4) what the probable result will be, and
   (5) how to evaluate the level of competency attainment (where such is possible).

The teaching and learning process employed by the instructor is designed to include a variety of laboratory experiences. In addition to standard lecture and discussion techniques, it is assumed that the instructor will include other learning devices available such as:

   (1) the case method,
   (2) role-playing,
   (3) independent study,
   (4) interaction with a personal computer,
   (5) elementary theory formulation,
   (6) response to questionnaires and self-testing devices,
   (7) individual projects,
   (8) small discussion groups, etc.

When there is time available, the instructor may wish to introduce action or applied research-based on independent investigation (e.g., descriptive research, game theory, debates, internship experiences, panels, forums).

Basically a three-step learning process is recommended. It should involve:

   (1) understanding of the objective of the learning experience module,
   (2) reading and comprehension of a "knowledge statement" or "lecturette" about the particular competency involved, and
   (3) skill learning or competency achievement through analysis and practice.

As the process proceeds, the instructor should:

    (1) assess initial student status,
    (2) introduce selected experiences to strengthen areas
        of weakness, and
    (3) evaluate competency attainment.

Based on literature analysis and responses from knowledgeable colleagues, the authors decided to offer a lengthy, but understandably incomplete listing of competencies and skills from the five areas determined. Primary competencies were selected from each of the five areas and were considered to be a practical number to include. They were categorized according to:

    (1) understandings developed,
    (2) skills acquired,
    (3) assessments carried out,
    (4) plans devised,
    (5) experiments undertaken,
    (6) evaluations made,
    (7) instruments employed, etc.

What then, most specifically, are these desirable management competencies or skills that were deemed most important at this point?

1. The Manager's Personal Competencies/Skills (selected from a list including 22 additional competencies/skills)

    a. Determine one's personal philosophy of life and/or religion
    b. Establish priorities in personal values clarification
    c. Develop a personal mission statement
    d. Develop a plan that (tentatively) maps out one's future (i.e., goal-setting in relation to maturity)
    e. Conduct a personal analysis to assist in the development of an individual time-management

plan (i.e., planning a work schedule for the week, month, year, etc.)

2. The Manager's Interpersonal Competencies/Skills (selected from a list including 24 additional competencies/skills)

   f. Develop an understanding of self (i.e., self-concept) as required for successful interpersonal competency
   g. Assess interpersonal communication skills (e.g., empathetic listening and responding)
   h. Execute an interpersonal style inventory
   i. Evaluate interpersonal management skills (e.g., selling ideas)
   j. Learn about one's leadership attributes and effectiveness; assess present leadership style

3. The Manager's Conceptual Competencies/Skills (selected from a list including 23 additional competencies/skills)

   k. Understand the development of twentieth century management thought, theory, and process
   l. Analyze the general (external) and immediate (internal) environments
   m. Develop an understanding of that phase of the management process generally known as PLANNING
   n. Develop an understanding of that phase of the management process generally known as ORGANIZING.
   o. Develop an understanding of that phase of the management process generally known as STAFFING
   p. Develop an understanding of that phase of the management process known as DIRECTING
   q. Develop an understanding of that phase of the management process known as

117

CONTROLLING

r. **Develop an understanding of a systems approach to the overall management process**

4. **The Manager's Technical Competencies/Skills (selected from a list including 36 additional competencies/skills)**

s. **Learn how to use the meeting as an effective tool for the work group.**
t. **Learn about team-building (i.e., developing an understanding of how work groups are formed and maintained.**
u. **Execute an in-basket analysis as the manager approaches a day on the job**
v. **Understand legal liability in relation to sport management**

Note: The above technical competencies/skills were selected from a total of 36 competencies and skills.

5. **The Manager's Conjoined Competencies/Skills (selected from a list including a total of 18 competencies/skills)**

w. **Develop an outline of a policies and procedures manual for a special event (e.g., a sports tournament).**
x. **Develop an approach to decision-making in relation to one's personal and professional philosophy (including ethical decision-making where applicable).**
y. **Carry out a strategic market-planning assessment for a sport and/or physical activity-based program.**
z. **Understand how to manage for change.**

Successful Student Should Demonstrate Achievement
in Representative Number of Competencies/Skills

Obviously there is insufficient time in any one undergraduate course in *any* of the proposed areas in the professional curriculum for physical activity education. However, whatever the situation may be, including the length and extent of the course experience (i.e., quarter, term, or semester), the successful student should demonstrate achievement and/or completion of at least a *representative sampling* of the competencies/skills deemed necessary in each of the eight areas (e.g., functional effects of physical activity, socio-cultural foundations of developmental physical activity) for eventual awarding of the baccalaureate degree.

Since a "competency-development approach" has not been used fully previously in the field except possibly to a limited extent in selected courses, some problems may arise regarding what shape or form the completed "laboratory reports" should assume in the various courses included in the curriculum. Each instructor will necessarily have to experiment with the laboratory phase of the course in question. Recommendations for time involvement and other expectations for actual student involvement in written reports and analyses will be needed. The instructor, based on ongoing experience and student evaluation, has to decide how much time will be allotted to lectures and how much laboratory experience will be offered. In addition to the occasional quiz, the instructor and/or a teaching assistant will have a set of exercises to correct with each "laboratory report" submitted. Also, there would normally be some sort of a "knowledge final" based on the course material included. It would probably be best for both the instructor and student to hand in each set of laboratory experiences by specified dates throughout the semester.

Concluding Statement

In this analysis the investigator argued that physical education, as a field of endeavor within educational institutions, has gradually but steadily declined in the second half of the twentieth century. The question was asked rhetorically whether physical education per se can ever achieve the aims and objectives envisioned by its leaders in the first half of the twentieth century. Indeed, can the field of physical education ever hope to become vital to the provision of healthful, developmental physical activity for all of the country's population whether these people are students or members of the general public?

This question should be answered in the affirmative--i.e., the field could become a full-fledged subject matter if the present field of physical activity education and educational sport (or sport and physical education as called within NASPE) were to make a number of changes in its present modus operandi. These recommended changes are as follows:

1. That the *field* be called physical activity education,
2. That the under girding *discipline* be called kinesiology,
3. That professional practitioners be known as *physical activity educators*,
4. That physical activity educators adopt a broadly based, consensual model for the body of knowledge and the competencies/skills required for their endeavors as professional educators,
5. That *professional literacy* for the practitioner be defined as the expert knowledge and competency desired for the physical activity educator,

(Note: Such professional literacy is over and above the concept of *cultural literacy* prescribed by Hirsch.)

6. That the physical activity educator should steadily become known more as *a specialist in human physical activity in exercise, sport, and related physical activity*,
7. That physical activity educators should promote more vigorously their own their own field of *physical activity education* and their own *discipline* of kinesiology.

(Not: The intent here is that use of terms and names identified primarily with other disciplines and professions should be avoided to the greatest possible extent [e.g., physiology of

120

exercise instead of physical activity science, sociology of sport instead of socio-cultural aspects of physical activity].)

8. That physical activity educators should become experts in their own *self-described* field,

(Note; This means a departure from the present "jack-of-all-trades, master-of-none" image now held. A thoroughgoing competency-development approach should be instituted in all professional preparation programs for physical activity educators prior to the awarding of the academic degree.)

9. That the profession, employing a systems approach, needs to develop an evolving online inventory of scientific findings about kinesiology that is categorized and arranged as ordered generalizations for daily use by the professional practitioner,

10. *That to accomplish the ultimate professional goal, involvement with competitive sport as a coach should be separated from the duties of the physical activity educator in the educational environment,* and

11. That the educational efforts of the physical activity educator should be extended to serve people on a lifelong basis in society at large.

(Note: This would involve licensing and/or certification for such public professional practice.)

Such a halcyon state, one that is still possible in the foreseeable future, could be achieved if the established professional association and those responsible for professional preparation in colleges and universities could become ready for such a development. The challenge is to guide qualified and deeply motivated professional students to full literacy in a discipline called kinesiology, while at the same time preparing them professionally also to a high standard in physical activity education. If this were to become the norm, and these graduates were imbued with a life purpose to provide people of all ages and conditions with purposeful, developmental physical activity, physical activity educators could indeed create a nation of healthy, vigorous people that would set an example for the world.

References

Adelman, M. (1971). A bibliography of master's and doctoral studies related to the history of sport and athletics in the United States (1930-1967). In E. F. Zeigler, M. L. Howell, & M. Trekell (Eds. & Aus.), *Research in the history, philosophy, and international aspects of physical education and sport: Bibliographies and techniques* (pp. 131-161). Champaign, IL: Stipes.

Berelson, B., & Steiner, G.A. (1964). *Human behavior.* NY: Harcourt, Brace, Jovanovich. *ENCARTA World English Dictionary.* (1999). NY: St. Martin's Press.

Hirsch, E. D., Jr., Kett, J, F., & Trefil, J. (1991). *The dictionary of cultural literacy.* Boston: Houghton Mifflin.

Katz, R. L. (Sept.-Oct., 1974). Skills of an effective administrator. *Harvard Business Review,* 51, 5:90-102.

Newell, K.M. (Dec, 1990). Physical education in higher education: Chaos out of order. *Quest,* 42, 1:227-242.

Siedentop, D. (Dec. 1880). Commentary: The world according to Newell. *Quest, 42, 1:315-322.*

Snyder, R. A., & Scott, H. A. (1954). *Professional preparation in health, physical education, and recreation.* NY: McGraw-Hill.

Zeigler, E. F. (1962). A history of undergraduate professional preparation for physical education in the United States (1861-1961). In E. F. Zeigler (Ed.) *A history of physical education and sport in the United States and Canada* (pp. 225-253). Champaigm, IL: Stipes. (This was originally published in 1962 as a background chapter in a national conference of professional preparation sponsored by the AAHPER, Washington, DC.)

Zeigler, E. F. (1982). *Physical education and sport: An introduction.* Philadelphia: Lea & Febiger.

Zeigler, E. F. (1990). *Sport and physical education: Past, present, future.* Champaign, IL: Stipes.

Zeigler, E. F. & Bowie, G. W. (1995). *Management competency development in sport and physical education.* Champaign, IL: Stipes.

Zeigler, E. F. (1997). From one image to a sharper one. *The Physical Educator,* 54, 1: 1-6.

PART 5
Sport Management Must Show Social Concern
As It Develops Tenable Theory

Today sport and all other social institutions (e.g., religion, politics, economics) are confronted with the need to demonstrate that they are worthwhile and responsible. Sport managers should truly understand what sport's status is, and how and why sport such standing occurred. Difficult decisions, often ethical in nature, will have to be made as the members of the sport management societies worldwide strive to continue the development of this profession/discipline. These professionals need to decide to what extent they wish to live up to the broad ideals of the programs being promoted by public, semipublic, or private agencies for all types of people of all ages. Those involved with professional preparation and scholarly endeavor urgently need a theory and a disciplinary model to place professional preparation for administrative or managerial leadership within the field on a gradually improving, sound academic basis. Practitioners need an online service that provides them with scholarly applied findings as they seek to serve in the behaviorally oriented environment of today's world.

An epoch in civilization approaches closure when many of the fundamental convictions of its advocates are challenged by a substantive minority of the populace. It can be argued that indeed the world is moving into a new epoch as the proponents of postmodernism have been affirming over recent decades. Within such a milieu there are indications that the sport management profession is going to have great difficulty crossing this chasm, this so-called, postmodern divide (Zeigler, 2003, p. 93).

Nevertheless, there is no question but that sport has become recognized as one of humankind's fundamental social institutions. However, I believe that there are now strong indications that sport's presumed overall recreational, educational, and entertainment role in the "adventure of civilization" is not being fulfilled adequately and certainly not most properly. Municipal recreation programs, private sport clubs, and school sport programs are "doing the best that they can" often with limited funding. At the same time the commercialized sport establishment gets almost all of the media attention and is prospering as never before. Thus, an intelligent, concerned citizen can reasonably ask, "What evidence do we have that sport as a social institution is really making a positive contribution to society?" I find myself forced to ask whether commercially organized sport is actually "talking a better game than it plays." Where or what is sport management's tenable theory? Recalling the well-known fairy tale. I find that I must declare--not that "the king doesn't have any clothes on"--but that "The king should prove (to society) that he is sufficiently clothed to justify our continuing support."

The sport industry is obviously "charging ahead" driven by capitalistic economic theory that overemphasizes ever-increasing gate receipts with an accompanying corollary of winning fueled somehow by related violence. One of the "principal principles" of physical education espoused in the early 1950s by Dr. Arthur Steinhaus (George Williams College) was that "sport was made for man, not man for sport"(1952). It is being countermanded day by day, week by week at all levels around the world. Interestingly, but disturbingly, a societal majority seems to lend support to this surge in the popularity of professionalized competitive sport. The athletes--those happy people on the way to the bank who do not mind being used as commodities--typically don't understand what is happening. They don't even recognize this as a problem. Neither do many (most?) aspiring sport management students in professional programs.

Everything considered, I am therefore forced to ask, "What are we helping to promote--we who have associated ourselves with sport management--and exactly why are we doing it?" I fear that we are simply going along with the seemingly inevitable tide. In the process we have become pawns to the prevailing sport establishment by "riding the wrong horse." Our present responsibility--to the extent that we are educators and scholars-- should be to devote our efforts to provide sport management with tenable theory. This tenable theory should relate to sport and physical activity involvement for all people of all ages in society be they normal, accelerated, or special in status.

Governmental agencies sponsoring "amateur" sport competition should be able to state in their relationship to sport that: if "such-and-such" is done with reasonable efficiency and effectiveness through the sponsorship of sporting activities, then "such-and-such" will (in all probability) result. Personnel in these same agencies are striving to do just this, but not necessarily in an acceptable way consonant with overall societal values. Instead of working assiduously for a "from-the-ground-up" development of young athletes in the hope that they would achieve relatively superior status eventually, they are proceeding in what might be called a fast-track approach. By that I mean that governments are focusing primarily on the recruitment and development of potentially elite athletes who somehow come to their attention, athletes whom they hope will bring fame and glory to their country. So, again, I ask, where is the evidence that organized sport's goal is based on tenable theory consonant with societal values that claim to promote the welfare of all?

I was heartened, however, by the number of publications in the *Journal of Sport Management* that discussed future directions in research. Frisby's EFZ Lecture (2005) , in referring to "The Good, The Bad, and The Ugly" strikes just the right note in her conclusion by urging a broadened outlook for sport management. Next Costa's study (2005) using Delphi technique provided excellent discussion based on the opinions of leaders in the field as to future directions. Concern was expressed about the ability to achieve the goals outlined (e.g., additional cross-discipline research) within our own discipline. Then, the entire "Expanding Horizons" issue offered interesting insights and approaches about research for consideration (2005). Finally, Chalip's analysis in his 2005 EFZ Lecture titled "Toward a distinctive sport management discipline," points us toward the achievement of "distinctive relevance" for our field. (This idea of a distinctive approach for a sport-management model strikes a resounding chord with me. Below I will seek to add a bit to the profession's consideration of this problem.)

Fortunately, also, there is a growing minority within the populace that supports a more humanistic position that accepts the steadily mounting evidence that all people--not just elite athletes striving for personal fulfillment and fame--need to be active in physical recreational activities throughout their entire lives. This leads me to inquire as to what role the professional sport management societies worldwide should play in the guidance of its members toward this end. Hopefully these men and women, serving as qualified professionals seeking the achievement of their society's most desirable values, will increasingly be in a position to assist sport and related physical activity to serve all people in our world society in the best possible way.

Before such a dream can become a reality, however, we need to dig deeply in our respective "cultural psyches" to begin to understand how society got itself in the presently questionable situation. Until at least the majority of people in our world's culture understand what has happened, what should be done, and what can be done, there is little hope for improvement in what I believe to be an increasingly untenable situation.

In retrospect, the 18th century in the Western world witnessed revolutionary thought that had caused it now to be known as the Age of Reason (or "enlightenment"). This outlook was based on ideals of truth, freedom, and reason for all humans. In the United States, however, the Enlightenment vision of Thomas Jefferson that promised political and social liberation was somehow "turned upside down." What happened in American life in the 19th century was that "progress" came to mean "technocratic progress." This was not the anticipated social progress for all people that was to be influenced by the inculcation of such values as justice, freedom, and self-fulfillment. These vital goals of a democratic political system were simply subjugated to the more immediate instrumental values. As Leo Marx explains, this technological advancement "became the fulcrum of the dominant American world view" (p. 5).

In the realm of physical (activity) education there was a "battle of the systems" of exercise and gymnastics that took place in the final quarter of the 20th century. However, it was the burgeoning interest in sport that permitted sport to infiltrate in the program of school physical education as sport skills. This type of experience was expanded further in (what was termed) extracurricular activity with team sports for the more highly skilled boys and girls. Earlier physical education programs, where available, as well as programs in wartime eras, undoubtedly stressed the concept of education "of the physical" more than the "roll-out-the-ball" approach so evident in physical education in subsequent decades. There was also the concept of "education through the physical" was also promoted to a degree by the educational progressivists influenced by Deweyan pragmatism. Typically this broader emphasis waned during periods of war and international unrest.

Careful historical analysis of this situation has led me to believe that the steady development of the social institution of competitive sport in the United States over the past 150 years has reached a crossroads (Zeigler, 2005, Chaps. XI & XII). If a claim can reasonably be made that organized sports may be doing as much harm as it does good can be made, I am forced to ask, "Where is the sport management theory needed to refute such a proposition?" In the United States especially, and in much of the remainder of the world, there is seemingly little awareness that such a negative contention about organized sport can be made. The developing world permits without question the increasing commercialization that has brought about sport's expansion and current gargantuan status. The conventional wisdom seems to be that "highly organized sport is good for people and our country. The more involvement an individual can have with sport, either actively or passively, the better he or she will be."

In the meantime, however, the vast majority of the population is getting inadequate involvement in regular, physical activity designed to help them live healthy, active, fulfilling lives. Many of these same people now possess--what Herbert Spencer in the mid-nineteenth century--called "seared physical consciences" He argued that in increasingly urbanized society there is inadequate physical activity education in the schools (1949). These same people simply don't know or appreciate what vigorous physical health "feels like." At the same time throughout their lives they are constantly being encouraged to pay increasing amounts of money to watch "skilled others" play games. (The resultant inactivity has created a crisis situation that will be discussed in some detail below.)

Hard Questions About Present Social Institutions

Social institutions are created and nurtured within a society ostensibly to further the positive development of the people living within that culture. Take democracy, for example, as a type of political institution that is currently being promoted vigorously by the United States throughout the entire world. (Such worldwide change will take time!) Within this form of social development, democracy has "struck up a deep relationship with economics and has found an eager bedfellow with whom to associate"--i.e., the institution of capitalism. Economics, of course, is another vital social institution upon which a society depends fundamentally. As world civilization developed, a great many of the world's countries have enacted with almost messianic zeal the promotion of such social institutions as democracy, capitalism, and --now!-- an increasing involvement with competitive sport. The "theory" is that the addition of highly competitive sport to this mix will bring about more "good" than "bad" for the countries involved. But has it? Disturbing questions have now begun to arise in various quarters.

What does this mean as we move along in the 21st century? Think of the example being set in North America, for example. Is there reasonable hope that the present brand of "combined" democratic capitalism that uses up the world's environmental resources inordinately will somehow improve the world situation in the long run? Can we truly claim with any degree of certainty that this "mix" of democracy and capitalism (with its subsequent inclusion of big-time sport) is producing more "good" than "bad"? (Admittedly, we do need to delineate between "what's 'good'" and "what's 'bad'" more carefully) There is no escaping the fact that the gap economically between the rich and the poor is steadily increasing. This means that "the American dream for all" is beginning to look like a desert mirage. Will the historical "Enlightenment Ideal" remain as an unfulfilled dream forever?

One of the results of the increasing development of the social institution of competitive sport is the creation of sport management societies in the respective regions and countries where such expansion has occurred. At the same time the question may be asked whether this development has reached a point where a claim can be made that highly competitive sport as a social phenomenon may be doing more harm than good in society. It is not that competitive sport does not have the potential for good that is being questioned here. (The world seems to have accepted this as fact!) It's the way that it is being carried out that is the problem. The world community does not really know whether this contention is true or not. Yet sport's expansion is permitted and encouraged almost without question in all quarters. "Sport is good for people, and more involvement with sport of almost any type--extreme sport, professional wrestling--is better" seems to be the conventional wisdom. Witness, also, the millions of dollars that are being parceled out of tax revenues for the several Olympic enterprises perennially. So long as it's thought that "a buck's to be made," also, permit even Evander Holyfield to box professionally in what's called a sport until he won't be able to remember his own name!

In the meantime, the large majority of the population in the developed world is getting inadequate involvement in physical activity, with obesity increasing unduly at all ages and levels. This is a highly significant problem that is increasing daily. Conversely there is rampant starvation in the underdeveloped world where most people, including children, must labor inordinately just to survive. At the same time the public in the technologically developed world is being expected to pay increasing amounts of money to watch "skilled others," either on television or "in the flesh," play types of games and sports increasing in complexity and danger almost exponentially. At the same time, "The National Institutes of Health estimates that Americans will take five years off the average life span," reports Randolph in "The Big, Fat American Kid Crisis" (*The New York Times*, 2006). The eventual outcome of what is happening today can be encapsulated in the grim predictions that the bulk of children and youth in the coming generation of the developed world may be the first to die before their parents because of obesity, less physical activity, and related health problems.

Resultantly, I am forced to ask "What really are we promoting, and do we know why are we doing it?" I do not have a complete answer to these questions, of course. But I do believe this strongly: we need to develop a theory of sport that will permit us to assess whether what we call "competitive sport" is fulfilling its presumed function of promoting good in a society. To do this. we will need to establish connections and relationships with a variety of disciplines in the academic world. Some that come to mind immediately are sport sociology, sport history, sport psychology, sport philosophy, sport economics, as well as selected other fields where research findings could well have application to sport and related physical activity. Some of these fields are anthropology, social geography, and political science--all academic fields that could well be helpful in any assessment of the findings of sport management.

I want to emphasize, also, that the field of sport management must keep a healthy balance between the theoretical and the practical in its ongoing scholarship and research. To do otherwise would be courting the same fate that befell the former Philosophic Society for the Study of Sport (now the IAPS). I'm sad to report that sport philosophy "went disciplinary" in the late 1960s and only recently on occasion has it descended from that lofty perch. As the third president of the Society, my warning on this point in 1975 was to no avail (Zeigler, 1976). Today the International Association for Sport Philosophy has a limited number of members and "they speak to no one," relatively speaking, except each other on occasion. This is an outcome that the field sport management will need to guard against assiduously. (Nevertheless, the disciplinary aspects of sport management should be pursued diligently, but there must be an accompanying pragmatic emphasis on applied research that is regularly and consistently downloaded to the "real world" where sport in its many forms takes place daily.)

Sport should be conducted in its various settings now and in the future, both generally and specifically, in a manner that will encourage its proper professional, educational and recreational uses, as well as its semiprofessional and professional concerns To guarantee such a state of affairs, sport must be challenged on an ongoing basis by people at all levels in a variety of ways. If this were to be the case, sport might possibly regain and retain those aspects that can contribute significant value to individual and social living.

In making these assertions, I must first define my terms accurately so that you are fully aware of what I am seeking to explain and also critique here. This is necessary because the term "sport," based on both everyday usage and dictionary definition, still exhibits radical ambiguity. Such indecision undoubtedly adds to the present confusion. So, when the word "sport" is used here, it will refer--unless indicated otherwise--to "competitive physical activity, an individual or group competitive activity involving physical exertion or skill, governed by rules, and sometimes engaged in professionally" (*Encarta World English Dictionary*, 1999, p. 1730).

Analyzing Sport's Role in Society

In this process of critiquing competitive sport, I believe further that society should strive to keep sport's drawbacks and/or excesses in check to the greatest possible extent. In recent decades we have witnessed the rise of sport throughout the land to the status of a fundamentalist religion. For example, we find sport being called upon to serve as a redeemer of wayward youth, but-- as it is occurring elsewhere--it is also becoming a destroyer of certain fundamental values of individual and social life.

Wilcox (1991), for example, in his empirical analysis, challenged "the widely held notion that sport can fulfill an important role in the development of national character." He stated that "the assumption that sport is conducive to the development of positive human values, or the 'building of character,' should be viewed more as a belief rather than as a fact." He concluded that his study did "provide some evidence to support a relationship between participation in sport and the ranking of human values" (pp. 3, 17, 18, respectively).

Assuming Wilcox's view has reasonable validity, those involved in any way in the institution of sport--if they all together may be considered a collectivity--should contribute a quantity of redeeming social value to our North American culture, not to mention the overall world culture (i.e., a quantity of good leading to improved societal well-being). On the basis of this argument, the following questions are postulated initially for possible subsequent response by concerned agencies and individuals (e.g., federal governments, state and provincial officials, philosophers in the discipline and related professions):

(1) Can, does, or should a great (i.e., leading) nation produce great sport?

(2) With the world being threatened environmentally in a variety of ways, should we now be considering an "ecology" of sport in which the beneficial and disadvantageous aspects of a particular sporting activity are studied through the endeavors of scholars in other disciplines as well?

(3) If it is indeed the case that the guardian of the "functional satisfaction" resulting from sport is (a) the sports person, (b) the spectator, (c) the businessperson who gains monetarily, (d) the sport manager, and, in some instances, (e) educational administrators and their respective governing boards, then who in society should be in a position to be the most knowledgeable about the immediate objectives and long range aims of sport and related physical activity?

(4) If the answer to question No.3 immediately above is that this person should be the trained sport and physical activity management professor, is it too much of a leap to also expect that person's professional association (!) to work to achieve consensus about what sport and closely related physical activity should accomplish? Further, should the professional association have some responsibility as the guardian (or at least the assessor) of

whether the aforementioned aims and objectives are being approximated to a greater or lesser degree?

Answering these questions is a truly complex matter. First, as I have stated above, sport and related physical activity have become an extremely powerful social force in society. Secondly, if we grant that sport now has significant power in all world cultures--a power indeed that appears to be growing--we should also recognize that any such social force affecting society can be dangerous if perverted (e.g., through an excess of nationalism or commercialism). With this in mind, I am arguing further that sport has somehow achieved such status as a powerful societal institution without an adequately defined underlying theory. Somehow, most of countries seem to be proceeding generally on a typically unstated assumption that "sport is a good thing for society to encourage, and more sport is even better!" And yet, as explained above, the term "sport" still exhibits radical ambiguity based on both everyday usage and dictionary definition. This obviously adds even more to the present problem and accompanying confusion.)

As we delve into this matter more seriously, we may be surprised--or perhaps not. We may well learn that sport is contributing significantly in the development of what are regarded as the *social* values--that is, the values of teamwork, loyalty, self-sacrifice, and perseverance consonant with prevailing corporate capitalism in democracy and in other political systems as well. Conversely, however, we may also discover that there is now a great deal of evidence that sport may be developing an ideal that opposes the fundamental moral virtues of honesty, fairness, and responsibility in the innumerable competitive experiences provided (Lumpkin, Stoll, and Beller, 1999).

Significant to this discussion are the results of investigations carried out by Hahm, Stoll, Beller, Rudd, and others in recent years. The Hahm-Beller Choice Inventory (HBVCI) has now been administered to athletes at different levels in a variety of venues. It demonstrates conclusively that athletes will not support what is considered "the moral ideal" in competition. As Stoll and Beller (1998) see it, for example, an athlete with moral character demonstrates the moral character traits of honesty, fair play, respect, and responsibility whether an official is present to enforce the rules or not. This finding was further substantiated by Priest, Krause, and Beach (1999) who reported that their findings changes over a four-year period in a college athlete's ethical value choices were consistent with other investigations. They showed decreases in "sportsmanship orientation" and an increase in "professional" attitudes associated with sport.

On the other hand, even though dictionaries define social character similarly, sport practitioners, including participants, coaches, parents, and officials, have come to believe that character is defined properly by such values as self-sacrifice, teamwork, loyalty, and perseverance. The common expression in competitive sport is: "He/she showed character"--meaning "He/she 'hung in there' to the bitter end!" [or whatever]. Rudd (1999) confirmed that coaches explained character as "work ethic and commitment." This coincides with what sport sociologists have found. Sage (1998. p. 614) explained that "Mottoes and slogans such as 'sports builds character' must be seen in the light of their ideological issues" In other words, competitive sport is structured by the nature of the society in which it occurs. This would appear to mean that over-commercialization, drug-taking, cheating, bribe-taking by officials, violence, etc. at all levels of sport are simply reflections of the culture in which we live. Where does that leave us today as we consider sport's presumed relationship with moral character development?

This discussion about whether sport's presumed educational and recreational roles have justification in fact could go on indefinitely. So many negative incidents have occurred that one hardly knows where to turn to avoid further negative examples. On the one hand we read the almost unbelievably high standards stated in the Code of Conduct developed by the Coaches Council of the National Association for Sport and Physical Education (2001). Conversely we learn that today athletes' concern for the presence of moral values in sport declines over the course of a university career (Priest, Krause, and Beach, 1999).

With this as a backdrop, we learn further that Americans, for example, are increasingly facing the cost and consequences of sedentary living (Booth & Chakravarthy, 2002). Additionally, Malina (2001) tells us that there is a need to track people's involvement in physical activity and sport across their life spans. Finally, Corbin and Pangrazi (2001) explain that we haven't yet been able to devise and accept a uniform definition of wellness for all people. The one thought that emerges from these various assessments is as follows: We give every evidence of wanting our "sport spectaculars" for the few much more than we want all people of all ages and all conditions to have meaningful sport and exercise involvement throughout their lives.

Sport Management Theory and Practice

Defined traditionally, we might say that the sport manager is one who plans, organizes, staffs, leads (or directs), and controls (i.e., monitors and evaluates) progress toward predetermined goals within programs of sport for people of all ages, be they in normal, accelerated, or special populations. To place the current topic in historical perspective (i.e., the beginning of investigation about the management [or administration] of sport and physical activity in educational institutions largely), master's and doctoral degrees about the subject within departments and schools of education in the United States were completed initially at Columbia Teachers College and New York University starting in the mid-1920s. Individually, there were many well-intended, seemingly worthwhile studies completed. However, it was impossible to say what these--literally--thousands of investigations "added up to" 35 years later at the beginning of the 1960s decade was really not known.

In the 1960s, however, research and scholarship in administrative theory and practice related to physical education and athletic administration began to receive attention in several quarters. Through the efforts of King McCristal (dean) and the author (University of Illinois, U-C), we were able to get this area included as one of six subject-matter areas in the Big Ten Body-of-Knowledge Project. In the fall of 1972, a symposium was held on the subject at The University of Michigan, Ann Arbor. In a volume published in 1975, the results of 20 doctoral dissertations carried out at Illinois were published (Zeigler and Spaeth, 1975). However, financial and other constraints in higher education of the 1970s slowed this development down considerably.

Then the rise of a so-called disciplinary approach to the field of physical education, plus the perennial claim of the "educational essentialist" that it is only the hard sciences that provide the basic knowledge, resulted in the introduction of the term kinesiology to supplement (or even supplant!) that of physical education at the university level. This tended to severely downgrade the importance of administrative theory and practice programs within the field, while job opportunities for professors related to biomechanics, exercise physiology, and motor learning increased. Concurrently, however, burgeoning interest in commercialized, highly competitive sport within higher education and in the public sector created a need for the establishment and development of college and university curricula in sport management. So the essence of what was often being eliminated in one program appeared to be springing up in a new curriculum stream--sport management. It was at this point on February 24, 1986 that a small group of us witnessed the successful creation of the now-successful North American Society for Sport Management.

Most of those behind the establishment of NASSM actually envisioned an association with a broad emphasis leading to the promotion of sport and physical activity for all people of all ages. However, interest in highly organized, elite sport seems to have engulfed conference presentations in the various aspects of competitive sport management. Sport management has rapidly become a mushrooming field in its own right that increasingly has its own curriculum independent of former physical education and athletics administration courses in educational institutions. Concurrently, the "eager scientists" in kinesiology, who conceptually relegated administrative theory and practice for physical education and athletics to the dustbin insofar as its place in their disciplinary curriculum is concerned, are presumably now quite happy and relieved in those sites where such separation has actually occurred.

Intramural and recreational sport is actually doing quite well at the college and university level, but is almost nonexistent at the high-school level and lower. Finally, the near demise of physical activity programs "for the many"--required within education at all levels within education prior to 1950--does not even appear on the radar screen of the large majority of professional preparation personnel in universities. Yet, because of the decline of required physical education, it has become starkly apparent that the health and physical fitness of the populace needs a strong shot in the arm to again establish a firm foothold in public consciousness. (It doesn't seem that the "War on Terrorism" will bring this change. Do we need another world war to accomplish this?) This is true even though--almost daily--reports of scientific studies tell us of the beneficial effects of regular physical activity on the human organism in so many different ways.

In such a developing world environment, then, what is the mission of a field called sport management, still a fledgling profession but one that is rapidly catching on all over the world? Frankly, I believe strongly that our profession needs to understand (define?) its mission much better than appears to be the case at present. Exactly what is its fundamental purpose in society? Further, how does the mission of sport management globally relate to the mission of the various professional associations composed primarily of men and women involved in the professional education of future sport managers? (Keep in mind that the typical professional sport promoters worldwide presently live in "another world"!)

Unfortunately, as I see it, the outlooks or aims of those people who today promote sport competition professionally, and that of those who believe they are promoting such competition educationally, appear to be getting closer all the time. I am referring here to the people involved, for example, in the National Basketball Association or the National Collegiate Athletic Association in the United States, respectively. Granted that the people in both of these associations are operating on the assumption that the provision of highly competitive sport opportunities in society is a good thing. Also, they appear to believe that promoting ever more opportunity for the masses to observe such activity is worthwhile. The fact that the cultivation of a "fan club" for professional sport also provides exorbitant income for the "accelerated few" athletes and a dubious future for the vast majority of athletes who don't "make it" appears to be of little concern. This is unfortunate for that "vast majority" because their educational background has typically been stunted by excessive involvement in competitive sport while enrolled at universities.

Frankly, I believe this assumption of "goodness " for society has become a dubious premise or principle upon which most of these promoters and/or educational administrators are operating. I maintain that this is so unless they can provide accompanying evidence to substantiate to society that the continuation and enlargement of the present trend to increasing commercialization in sport is contributing positively to society as a social institution. To repeat, all social institutions must have an underlying theory to justify their continuing existence. The basic question, I submit, is simply this: In this evolving situation, what kind of "good"--philosophically speaking--can we claim is currently being created by competitive sport?

To one who has followed and written extensively about this development down through the 20th century from both a historical and a philosophical standpoint, I can only report (sadly!) that the excesses and corruption of competitive sport have increased steadily decade by decade. And, even more sadly, the seemingly jaded public (as fans) does not seem to realize--or seems to accept--that sport's status as a desirable social institution is being lowered steadily with each passing year. (I won't even get into the question of the taking of one or more of 400-500 drugs to enhance performance that the sport establishment is facing today.) Competitive sport is forced to stay within the law, but its typically laudable creed espoused so freely requires an enforceable code of ethics in the present--not as a dream for the future.

Concurrently, the low status perennially accorded to physical education-except in times of war when referred to as "physical fitness"-continues. This is true even though ongoing research in kinesiology and physical education--and the field's related disciplines--is steadily making the case for regular, developmental physical activity as an essential, if not a vital, social institution to be employed for the benefit of all. Nevertheless the term "sport," and what it connotes to the average mind, largely overrides the need for the provision of necessary funding of developmental physical activity as a social institution. I firmly believe that provision for the managing and promoting developmental physical activity in sport, exercise, and physical recreation for people of all ages, be they part of accelerated, normal, or special populations, should at least be an auxiliary part of our mission in sport management. Yet we find that our professional associations and disciplinary societies relayed to "physical activity" are steadily and increasingly becoming more disjointed as they grow farther apart. Other professions and disciplines are "filling in" where we should be "producing" (e.g., recreation, medicine).

You can see where I am heading with this analysis. I believe it is now incumbent upon the field of sport management (i.e., these professional organizations worldwide) to investigate and subsequently understand precisely what effect sport, however defined and with all of its ramifications, is having on society. Is it more good than bad? Who knows? The professional and semiprofessional sport managers can't answer this basic question. (Many probably wouldn't want to know anyhow if it meant a possible shifting of emphasis in their offerings.) Therefore I urge the world's various professional sport management associations to take a hard look at what appears to be a steadily growing problem. They need to determine (1) what effect sport is having on society; (2) if there is a problem with the present development, and to what extent the professional associations (e.g., in North America) may unwittingly be part of the problem; and (3) in what ways professional sport management associations can ensure that sport as a whole, and more specifically its many programs at all levels, are moving in the right direction? These questions can't be answered satisfactorily without an underlying theory of sport management that meets the needs of all people.

Need for a Theory of Sport Management

Returning to the assertion made earlier, a theory underlying sport management could contribute greatly to the answering of the questions raised immediately above. It would need to be related basically to the social sciences and to certain professions that carry out their own independent research as well (e.g., business administration). It should contain "propositions of fact" that can, at least in principle, be verified empirically. "Propositions of value" are subjective and therefore typically conform to societal values and norms. Therefore, it would not be a philosophy of sport management, although a concerned individual or group might well philosophize about such human activity.

A theory is not a taxonomy, however, although a taxonomy of sport management will necessarily evolve as scientific and scholarly investigation about it is carried out. "A taxonomy may be defined as a classification of data according to their natural relationships, or the principles governing such classifications....In fact, one could probably make a good case to support the contention that any science begins with a taxonomy. . . ." (Griffiths, 1959. p. 17)

A Proposed Taxonomy for Sport Management.

Below as Table 2, I have included a sample of what a taxonomy of sport management might look like. It includes both scholarly and professional dimensions with three headings defined as (1) areas of scholarly study and research, (2) related disciplinary aspects, and (3) professional aspects. The possibility of "streaming" is mentioned at the undergraduate level. Also, there are three categories of graduate education postulated.

The development of a model, or taxonomy, could be important for evolving theory because it would enable a researcher not only to ask questions, but also to speculate as to how they might be answered. The term "model" has a number of

140

Table 2

UNDERGRADUATE CURRICULUM IN SPORT MANAGEMENT:

Areas of Scholarly Study & Research	Related Disciplinary Aspects	Professional Aspects
I. BACKGROUND, MEANING, & INTERCULTURAL SIGNIFICANCE	-History -Philosophy	-International Relations -Professional Ethics -International & Compar. Study
II. SOCIO-CULTURAL & BEHAVIORAL ASPECTS	-Sociology -Economics -Psychology (individ. & social) -Anthropology -Political Science -Geography -Law	-Application of Theory to Prac.
III SPORT MANAGEMENT THEORY	-Management Science - -Business Administration (e.g., sport marketing, -sport finance, facility management, sales)	-Application of Theory to Prac.
IV. CURRICULUM THEORY & PROGRAM DEVELOPMENT	-Curriculum Studies	-Application of Theory to Prac.

1. *General Education*: universities and colleges typically have a distribution requirement for all students in the humanities, social-science, and natural sciences.
2. *Professional* Core Subjects: an irreducible minimum requirement in the following subjects is required: communication & media relations, economic theory & sport finance, sport marketing, sponsorship & sales, legal aspects, sport governance, sport ethics, the international sport industry, and sport & physical activity internships.
3. *Specialized* Undergraduate Professional Preparation; streaming possibilities may be added in the degree program.
4. *Graduate* Education; three types of specialization are desirable: (1) professional preparation stream; (2) disciplinary stream, (3) practitioner stream)

V. MEASUREMENT & EVALUATION	-Theory about the - Measurement Function	-Application of to Theory & Practice.

141

meanings. The one that concerns a developing theory of sport management would be: "a description of a set of data in terms of a system of symbols, and the manipulation of the symbols according to the rules of the system. The resulting transformations are translated back into the language of the data, and the relationship discovered by the manipulations are compared with the empirical data." (Griffiths, p. 44)

Note here, however, the difficulty of "manipulating symbols" unless , for example, one is trying to explain anything other than present social developments. To seek to determine those that occurred in history, one would be well advised initially to attempt to estimate the strength of each conceivable influence that might have caused a past social occurrence or historical phenomenon.

By now governmental, educational, and commercial agencies and organizations should be able to argue convincingly that sport is a "relatively homogeneous substance" that can serve at least reasonably well as an indispensable balm or aid to human fulfillment within an individual life (adapted from Barzun [speaking about art], 1974, p. 12). However, the idea of "sport and developmental physical activity for all" on a lifelong basis continues to receive more "lip support" than actual investment based on the monetary input of government toward overall fitness and physical recreational involvement for the general population. Yet the logical argument that--through the process of total psycho-physical involvement--sport provides highly desirable "flow experience" may well be true. The question is "for whom does the bell toll?" (Csikszentmihalyi, 1993, p. 183).

Below you will find "A Model for Sport Management Development (Including a Competency-Based Approach)" (see Figure 1 below) This model is an effort to resolve the relationship between what has been called the disciplinary aspects and those aspects that have been designated as "professional" in nature. I have included five elements as the fundamental ones in a model that portrays the basic elements of the developing sport management profession.

Figure 1

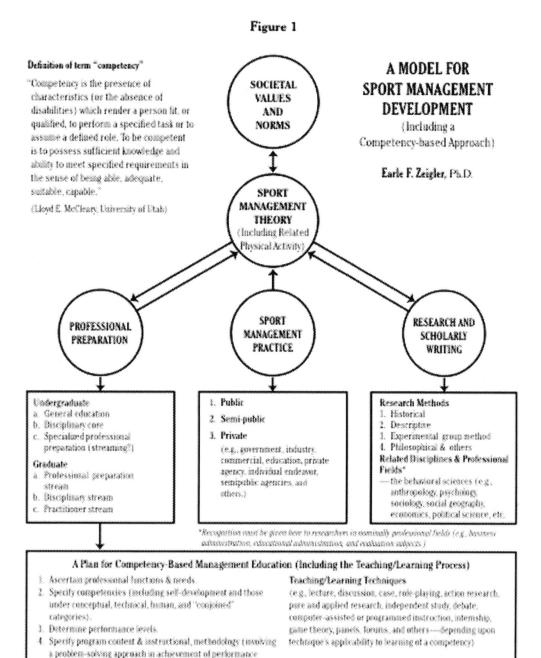

Definition of term "competency"

"Competency is the presence of characteristics (or the absence of disabilities) which render a person fit, or qualified, to perform a specified task or to assume a defined role. To be competent is to possess sufficient knowledge and ability to meet specified requirements in the sense of being able, adequate, suitable, capable."

(Lloyd E. McCleary, University of Utah)

SOCIETAL VALUES AND NORMS

A MODEL FOR SPORT MANAGEMENT DEVELOPMENT
(Including a Competency-based Approach)

Earle F. Zeigler, Ph.D.

SPORT MANAGEMENT THEORY
(Including Related Physical Activity)

PROFESSIONAL PREPARATION

SPORT MANAGEMENT PRACTICE

RESEARCH AND SCHOLARLY WRITING

Undergraduate
a. General education
b. Disciplinary core
c. Specialized professional preparation (streaming?)

Graduate
a. Professional preparation stream
b. Disciplinary stream
c. Practitioner stream

1. Public
2. Semi-public
3. Private
   (e.g., government, industry, commercial, education, private agency, individual endeavor, semipublic agencies, and others.)

Research Methods
1. Historical
2. Descriptive
3. Experimental group method
4. Philosophical & others

Related Disciplines & Professional Fields*
— the behavioral sciences (e.g., anthropology, psychology, sociology, social geography, economics, political science, etc.

*Recognition must be given here to researchers in nominally professional fields (e.g., business administration, educational administration, and evaluation subjects.)

A Plan for Competency-Based Management Education (Including the Teaching/Learning Process)

1. Ascertain professional functions & needs.
2. Specify competencies (including self-development and those under conceptual, technical, human, and "conjoined" categories).
3. Determine performance levels.
4. Specify program content & instructional methodology (involving a problem-solving approach in achievement of performance levels: what needs to be known; where obtained; organization of the learning experience; probable results, and others.
5. Identify and evaluate competency attainment.
6. Validate process periodically.

Teaching/Learning Techniques

(e.g., lecture, discussion, case, role-playing, action research, pure and applied research, independent study, debate, computer-assisted or programmed instruction, internship, game theory, panels, forums, and others——depending upon technique's applicability to learning of a competency)

(Adapted from McCleary & McIntyre 1973)

143

Note: As it happens, these elements also describe the basic elements of any profession [as I had suggested in the early 1970s for the field of management itself]; see Zeigler, 1972). Subsequently I incorporated the idea of competency and skill-acquisition into the model based on the recommendation by Lloyd McCleary, formerly of the University of Illinois, C-U. I subsequently realized that this entire model configuration fits very well into a description of the ongoing status of the sport-management profession.

The inclusion of "Societal Values & Norms" as an overarching entity in the model is based on the sociologic theory that the value system (i.e., the values and the norms) of a culture will be realized eventually within the society--if all goes well! Values represent the highest echelon of the social system level of the entire general action system. These values may be categorized into such "entities" as artistic values, educational values, social values, sport values, etc. Of course, all types or categories of values must be values held by personalities. The social values of a particular social system are those values that are conceived of as representative of the ideal general character that is desired by those who ultimately hold the power in the system being described. The most important social values in North America, for example, have been (1) the rule of law, (2) the socio-structural facilitation of individual achievement, and (3) the equality of opportunity (Johnson, 1994).

Norms--not to be confused with values--are the shared, sanctioned rules which govern the second level of the social structure. The average person finds it difficult to separate in his or her mind the concepts of values and norms. Keeping in mind the examples of values offered immediately above, some examples of norms are (1) the institution of private property, (2) private enterprise, (3) the monogamous, conjugal family, and (4) the separation of church and state.

Put simply, this means that decisions regarding the development of a profession are based on the prevailing values and norms over and above any scientific and/or scholarly evidence that may become available to strengthen existing theory.

Fundamentally, there is a hierarchy of control and conditioning that operates within the culture that exerts pressure downward affecting all aspects of the society. (Keep in mind that this pressure may be exerted upward as well.)

Moving downward from the top of Figure 1, the second phase of the model is called "Sport Management Theory." This is the systematic arrangement of proven facts or knowledge about a professional field (or discipline in the case of a subject-matter). From such theory we can also derive assumptions and testable hypotheses that should soon amplify as a result on ongoing scholarship, research, and experience. In the process scholars and researchers will also clarify a developing (and presumably) coherent group of general and specific propositions arranged as ordered generalizations) that can be used as principles of explanation for the phenomena that have been observed. Obviously, any profession must have a sound under girding body of knowledge if it hopes to survive with its professional status fully recognized in society. Unfortunately. at present there is no such inventory of scholarly and research findings about sport management theory readily available for those involved in sport management practice, professional preparation, and research and scholarly writing contributing to disciplinary development.

Moving downward once again, the model now expands both downward and to the right and left so that there is a total of three circles. In a sense these three circles would typically "feed" or "draw" knowledge and information from the middle circle above designated as "Sport Management Theory." Note that there are arrows going backward and forward in all directions to explain necessary "reciprocity" among these entities. These arrows show the complexity of the evolving subject.

The circle on the left is designated as "Professional Preparation." It includes the planned program designed to educate the professional practitioner. the teacher of practitioners. and--arguably--the scholar and/or researcher about the subject of professional preparation. The undergraduate program would presumably include (1) general education, (2) a disciplinary core, and (3) specialized professional preparation (conceivably with streaming possibilities). The graduate program could conceivably contain three distinct streams: (1) a professional-preparation stream; (2) a disciplinary stream. and (3) a practitioner stream.

The second of the three circles alongside each other in the upper half of the model is titled "Sport Management Practice." This would include those professional practitioners with degree programs involving general education, a sport management disciplinary-base, and specialized knowledge about the theory and practice of sport management in the range of public, semipublic, and private agencies and programs involved with varying types of sport and physical activity programs.

The third of the three circles (on the right) has been given the title of "Research and Scholarly Writing." Such research knowledge and scholarly writing is developed on an ongoing basis employing existing research methods and techniques to gather knowledge (i.e. propositions of fact) about the subject of sport management at all levels and under all conditions). Such research and scholarly writing is typically carried out by university professors and qualified professionals wherever employed. Obviously, there has been great--continuing!--help in the past provided by scholars and researchers in related disciplines and professional fields (e.g., the behavioral sciences and business administration).

The Next Step for the Sport Management Profession

Now that we have had a look at where sport management has been, and where it is currently, where should it go from here? The obvious answer would appear to be to build on--i.e., add scholarly sport management literature--to the available inventory of completed research on physical education and athletics management that has been made ready for entry into both departmental and personal data banks and/or retrieval systems by the efforts of scholarly people in the field since the mid-1920s. This historical literature has been delineated and recorded for sport and physical education management.

As it exists, it can be stored in such a way that an ongoing data base can be originated, maintained, and developed. To this should be added as soon as possible the results of investigations reported in the *Journal of Sport Management* and similar publications worldwide (e.g., the *International Journal of Sport Management*). This is the bare minimum that should be contemplated by professors or graduate students as they consider further research. They could at least determine what research has already been carried out on the particular topic at hand being considered for further research.

Despite the fact that this embryonic inventory of completed research is now available for easy storage and retrieval in a data base, what we have been able to accomplish with this data represents merely a "scratching of the surface." So much more needs to be done by our scholars in sport and related physical activity. Presently, dedicated practitioners for some time have been overwhelmed by periodical literature, monographs, and books from our field, from the allied professions, and from the related disciplines. Much of this information is interesting and valuable. However, it is so often not geared to the interests of professionals who are fulfilling many duties and responsibilities in the various positions they hold. Also, there is undoubtedly much overlapping material emanating also from the allied professions (notably recreation and park administration). Further, much of the available material--when a person by intent or chance happens to discover it--may be unintelligible, partially understandable, or not available in its essence and in a condensed form to the professional in sport management. Thus, one can only conjecture in what form such information will (or unfortunately won't) be conveyed to the many legislative or advisory boards on whose behalf we are carrying out our endeavor.

To make matters worse, because of provinciality and assorted communication barriers, our field is missing out on important findings now becoming available in Dutch, German, Japanese, Chinese, Italian, and the Scandinavian languages. Further, in addition to the above reason, because of a plethora of rules, regulations, and stipulations, people may not be receiving information about substantive reports of various government agencies at all levels. Such reports should become part of personal and departmental retrieval systems of those carrying out scholarly work in sub-disciplinary and sub-professional areas of investigation.

Interestingly, Joo and Jackson (2002) analyzed scholarly literature that had appeared in the *Journal of Sport Management* since its inception in 1987. Their analysis of 242 articles published showed that, although Trevor Slack's study in 1996 revealed that 65% of the published articles involved the delivery of either physical education or athletics programs, the emphases in research had shifted in the 1990s to marketing studies. More recently, however, there was a move to the area of organizational behavior. The results of research published in the *Journal of Sport Management,* as well as in the more recent *International Journal of Sport Management* should be entered into our bibliography and inventory as soon as possible. These findings should be correlated with studies reported as part of Zeigler's (1995) and Baker's (1983 and 1995) ongoing thesis and dissertation project with Collins and Zarriello, respectively. (Note: Contact author at <zeigrog@axion.net> to have bibliographic data from 1925-1972 downloaded.)

It is true that bibliographies of scholarly publications are occasionally made available. Further, printouts of bibliographies on specific concepts or uniterms can sometimes be purchased commercially. However, a bibliography is just that--a bibliography. Such a listing is typically not annotated to any degree, and one can hardly recall the last time a thorough bibliographical *commentary* on a topic related to sport management has been published.

The Most Important Point: The Need for an Ongoing Inventory. Still further--and this is really the most important point--it can be argued that the profession simply does not know where it stands in regard to the steadily developing body of knowledge in the many sub-disciplinary and sub-professional aspects of sport management (e.g., sport ethics, sport law, sport economics, sport marketing). Our profession--any profession for that matter!--needs such information as an inventory to form the basis--the theory, intellectual "underpinning," evidence, body of knowledge--for an evolving professional (practitioner's) handbook. In our case it would immediately become an essential component of every person's professional practice in the field of sport management. Nowhere does our professionals (and scholars, also) have such a steadily evolving "Inventory of Scholarly, Scientific Findings Arranged as Ordered Principles or Generalizations" in their hands (and also online) as an ever-evolving professional handbook to help them in their work daily--be they general manager, ticket manager, marketer, athletic director, head coach, management scholar or researcher, or whatever. Such information is obviously vitally important to the professional practitioner who could make use daily of the essence of this proposed "action-theory marriage." If such an inventory were to be made available, the profession should then carry such an inventory forward on a yearly, 2-, 3-, or 5-year basis of renewal for all practitioners in the profession. This deficiency can--and indeed must--be rectified as we move on into the 21st century.

Note: In 1985–more than 25 years ago!-this author began to make appeals to the executive and professional staff of the American Alliance for Health, Physical Education, Recreation, and Dance to engage in a project designed to make physical (activity) education's "body of knowledge" available to professional practitioners on-line. Although it was recognized that such a proposition was highly desirable, and a similar recommendation has been made periodically since that time, it was evidently felt that funding for such a project was not available.

Although the author has been discouraged about the fact that such an undertaking has never gotten underway through the efforts of the Alliance, the author nevertheless hasn't given up on what he considers now to be essential for the future of physical activity education. So, once again in 2010, the new executive vice-president of the Alliance was approached with this recommendation. Additionally, a similar recommendation has been made to the president and members of the Executive of the North American Society for Sport Management. The hope is that perhaps such an undertaking might be considered desirable and viable for this society. Accordingly, the essence of this plan is repeated below, this time with the profession of sport management only in mind.

Formulation of an Inventory of Scientific Findings. This recommendation to develop an inventory of scientific findings about sport management would not be unique to this field. Bernard Berelson and Gary Steiner (1964) postulated such an inventory 47 years ago in what they called the behavioral sciences. In their publication, *Human behavior: An inventory of scientific findings*, the editors and associates reported, integrated, assessed, and classified "the results of several decades of the scientific study of human behavior (p. 3). The basic plan of this formidable undertaking is fundamentally sound; thus, many of their ideas concerning format could be employed in the development of a scientific inventory of findings about sport management. Actually, it could well be carried out in all of the world's existing disciplines and then updated at regular intervals on a worldwide basis in one or more agreed-upon languages. Of course, varying emphases and certain significant differences might be introduced, but the basic approach is still valid. Berelson and Steiner summarized their task as the development of "important statements of proper generality for which there is some good amount of scientific evidence" (p. 5).

How the Inventory Would Be Constructed. The type of inventory recommended would develop through the combined effort of people in the various aspects of sport management and related disciplines and professions. The goal would be to present an inventory of knowledge on the subject of sport management-- that is, to assess the present state of knowledge and scholarly thought. Thus, those who prepare this information would be writing as reporters and knowledge-integrators, presenting what they know, and what they think they know, based on the available evidence. Every effort would have to be made to avoid presenting what they hope will be known. Down through the years there appear to have been frequent occasions in many professions where this latter approach has been followed, intentionally or otherwise, where people make declarative statements arguing that such thoughts are indeed based on documented evidence.

In such an inventory, the reader would find series of verified findings, principles and/or generalizations in an ordered 1-2-3-4 arrangement, typically with the citation of sources which generated the information. For example, several general theoretical propositions relative to "organizational behavior" could be considered according to several categories from Berelson and Steiner. The following findings about "The Organization," arranged as ordered generalizations, have been extracted from Berelson & Steiner (1964, pp. 365-373):

A1   The larger, the more complex, and the more heterogeneous the society, the greater the number of organizations and associations that exist in it.
   A1.1   Organizations tend to call forth organizations: If people organize on one side of an issue, their opponents will organize on the other side.
   A1.2   There is a tendency for voluntary associations to become more formal.
   A2   There is always a tendency for organizations (of a nonprofit character) to turn away, at least partially, from their original goals.
   A2.1 Day-to-day decisions of an organization tend to be taken as commitments and precedents, often beyond the scope for which they were initially intended, and thus they come to affect the character of the organization.

In reporting the available material, the language used should be as free as possible from scientific jargon. It should be understandable to the intelligent lay person and, of course, to professional practitioners in the area of sport and physical activity management. This would be difficult, because the findings would range from sport marketing to sport ethics to management competencies in a field that includes many areas of specialization. In any case, what would be presented is currently not available elsewhere in this form. This involves more than delineating by descriptive research technique what might be called "sport management literacy" (see, for example, Zeigler [1994] that presents "physical education and sport foundations" from which certain generalizations as explained above might be drawn). This type of inventory would represent a truly significant contribution to the profession of sport management, as well as the public for whose benefit sport is presumed to serve as a social institution.

To clarify this process further, the reader should understand that it may be necessary to select a particular study for inclusion in the inventory from among similar items available in the sport management literature--and also from among studies carried out in closely related fields (e.g., management science) that have a direct bearing on the major topic at hand The knowledge integrator or synthesizer (i.e. a *qualified* analyst) would be looking primarily for theory, findings, principles, generalizations, and propositions that apply to this field (i.e., the management of sport in its various forms worldwide). After accepting a finding for inclusion, it would be necessary to condense it and similar findings to one distinct principle or generalization. Next, the investigator would organize the material into subheadings that could subsequently be arranged in a logical, coherent, descending manner (e.g., Proposition A1, then A1.1, A1,1a, A1.1b, A1,1c, etc., depending upon the complexity of the proposition at hand). Finally, the resultant material would be reviewed and analyzed in order to eliminate certain technical language that might only confuse the majority of professionals for whom the inventory is primarily intended.

The goal of this project would be an inventory representing a distillation of the literature relating to the management of sport in all its forms, one that would communicate what scholars believe is known about the field to those professionals who are not specialists in the specific sub-disciplinary or sub-professional area described. This is not to say, of course, that such an inventory could not be helpful to the specialist in his or her own specialty. Further, to some extent there would at first be reliance on secondary summaries of the available literature, but this should be kept to a minimum. However, such reliance would be necessary because of the great bulk and variety of material. Also, the investigators could obtain the benefit of the evaluative judgment of the specialist who may have originally developed a summary or evaluation. Such material would be temporarily helpful in those instances where gaps in the field's own literature still exist (of which there are undoubtedly many).

Then, too, as more evidence is forthcoming, it would provide a base for improved professional operation as the fundamental and specialized management theory grows broader and deeper. Even then, the scholar, as well as the professional user of the generalized theory, would appreciate the necessity of using some qualifying statements in the development of ordered principles or generalizations (e.g., "under certain circumstances"). This inventory could be made available as an evolving professional handbook on the assumption that the steadily growing body of scientific findings about the management of developmental physical activity in sport and exercise is needed now by the many professionals in the field--be they managers, supervisors, teachers, coaches, or researchers in public, semipublic, or private agencies.

How This Inventory Would Be Constructed. The type of inventory recommended would develop through the combined effort of people in sport management, its allied professions, and its related disciplines (those that have any direct or tangential interest in the management of sport). The goal would be to present an inventory of knowledge on the subject of the management of sport and related physical activity--that is, to assess the present state of knowledge and scholarly thought. Thus, those who prepare this information would be writing as Reporters and Integrators presenting (1) what they know and (2) what they think they know based on the available evidence. (As mentioned above, every effort would have to be made to avoid presenting what they hope will be known.)

In such an inventory, the reader would find series of verified findings, principles and/or generalizations in an ordered 1-2-3-4 arrangement, typically with the Citation of Sources which generated the information. For example, the following general theoretical propositions relative to human behavior in managerial situations could be considered according to several categories (as adapted from Berelson and Steiner in the area of small-group research). The following theory relating to the athletic director in a university--that is, assumptions or testable hypotheses--might be included in an inventory:

1. That the manner in which the director of athletics leads his/her program is determined more by existing regulations of the educational institution itself, and the expectations of coaches and staff, than the manager's own personality and character traits.

2. That a director of athletics will find it most difficult to shift the department away from established norms.

3. That a director of athletics will receive gradually increasing support from coaches and staff members to the extent that he/she makes it possible for them to realize their personal goals.

4. That a director of athletics who attempts to employ democratic leadership will experience difficulty in reaching his/her own personal goals for the program if there are a significant number of authoritarian personalities in it (adapted from Berelson & Steiner, pp. 341-346).

Concluding Statement

In offering this perspective to the field of sport management, Daniel Wren's cautionary thought was in my mind. In the epilogue of his outstanding *History of Management Theory and Practice* (2005), he stated: "Management is more than an economic activity, however; it is a conceptual task that must mold resources into a proper alignment with the economic, technological, social, and political facets of its environment. We neglect the 'social facets' at our peril!"

It is these very "social facets" of the enterprise that the field of sport management needs to consider more carefully in the twenty-first century. Sport, as all other social institutions, is inevitably being confronted by the need to become truly responsible. Many troubling and difficult decisions, often ethical in nature, will have to be made as the professor of sport management continues the development of this profession/discipline as it seeks to prepare those who will guide sport in the years ahead. The fundamental question facing the profession is: "What *kind* of sport should the profession promote to help shape what sort of world in the 21st century? Professional sport management societies need to decide to what extent they wish to be involved with all types of sport for all types of people of all ages as they take part in healthful sport and physical activity promoted by public, semipublic, or private agencies.

There is no doubt but that the field of sport management made great strides in the closing years of the twentieth century. Nevertheless I believe that the field--both the profession and its related disciplinary effort--must develop underlying management thought, theory, and practice in an ongoing manner to support its professional practitioners. I stress again that practitioners "on the fire line" daily in sport management should be provided with an evolving inventory of ordered generalizations as to the best ways of carrying out their endeavor.

Finally, whatever decisions are made in regard to the future, we must continue to make all possible efforts to place professional preparation for administrative or managerial leadership within our field on a gradually improving, sound academic basis. The question of leadership confronts us from a number of different directions. Our field, and undoubtedly many others, desperately needs a continuing supply of first-class leaders. Any organization or enterprise soon begins to falter and even to stumble if it doesn't have good leadership. We should maintain our efforts to find more fine people who will take charge in the behaviorally oriented, sport management environment of today's world.

References

Baker, J. A. W. & Collins, M. S. (1983). *Research on administration of physical education and athletics 1971-1982*: A retrieval system. Reseda. CA: Mojave.

Baker, J. A. W. & Zarriello, J. (1995). *A bibliography of completed research and scholarly endeavor relating to management in the allied professions (1980-1990 inclusive)*. Champaign, IL: Stipes.

Barzun, Jacques. *The use and abuse of art*. Princeton: Princeton University Press, 1974, pp. 123-150.

Berelson, B., & Steiner, G. A. (1964). *Human behavior; An inventory of scientific findings*. New York: Harcourt, Brace & World.

Booth, F. W., & Chakravarthy, M. V. (2002). Cost and consequences of sedentary living: New battleground for an old enemy. *Research Digest (PCPFS)*, 3(16), 1-8.

Chalip, L. (2006). Toward a distinctive sport management discipline. *Journal of Sport Management*, 20(1), 1-22.

Corbin, C. B. & Pangrazi, R. P. (2001). Toward a uniform definition of wellness: A commentary. *President's Council on Physical Fitness and Sports Research Digest*. 3, 15, 1-8.

Costa, C. A. (2005). The status and future of sport management: A Delphi study. *Journal of Sport Management*, 19(2), 117-143.

Csikszentmihalyi, M. (1993), *The evolving self: A psychology for the third millennium*. NY: HarperCollins.

Encarta World English Dictionary, The. (1999). NY: St. Martin's Press.

Frisby, W. (2005). The good, the bad, and the ugly. *Journal of Sport Management*, 19(1), 1-12.

Griffiths, D. E. (1959) *Administrative Theory*. NY: Appleton-Century-Crofts.

Hahm, C.H., Beller, J. M., & Stoll, S. K. (1989). *The Hahm-Beller Values Choice Inventory*. Moscow, Idaho: Center for Ethics, The University of Idaho.

Johnson, H. M. (1994). Modern organizations in the Parsonsian theory of action. In A. Farazmand (Ed.), *Modern organizations: Administrative theory in contemporary society* (p. 59). Westport, CT: Praeger.

Joo, J. & Jackson, E. N. (2002). A content analysis of the Journal of Sport Management:: An analysis of sport management's premier body of knowledge.

Research Quarterly for Exercise and Sport, 73(1, Suppl.), A111.

Journal of Sport Management. (A special issue of the journal was devoted to the question of sport management research. Dated October, 2005, Vol. 19, No. 4 was titled "Expanding Horizons: Promoting Critical and Innovative Approaches to the Study of Sport Management".)

Kavussanu, M. & Roberts, G. C. (2001). Moral functioning in sport: An achievement goal perspective. *Journal of Sport and Exercise Psychology*, 23, 37-54.

Lumpkin, A., Stoll, S., & Beller, J. M. (1999). *Sport ethics: Applications for fair play* (2nd ed.). St. Louis, MO: McGraw-Hill.

Malina, R. M.. (2001). Tracking of physical activity across the life span. *Research Digest (PCPFS)*, 3-14, 1-8.

Marx, L. (1990). Does improved technology mean progress? In Teich, A. H. (Ed.),*Technology and the future*. NY: St. Martin's Press.

National Association for Sport and Physical Education. (2001). The coaches code of conduct. *Strategies*, 15(2), 11.

Priest, R. F., Krause, J. V., & Beach, J. (1999). Four-year changes in college athletes' ethical value choices in sports situations. *Research Quarterly for Exercise and Sport*, 70(1), 170-178.

Randolph, E. (2006). The big, fat American kid crisis…And 20 things we should do about it. *The New York Times*. (see http://select.nytimes.com/2006/05/10/opinion/10talkingpoints.html?pagewanted=all).

Rudd, A., Stoll, S. K., & Beller, J. M. (1999). Measuring moral and social character among a group of Division 1A college athletes, non-athletes, and ROTC military students. *Research Quarterly for Exercise and Sport*, 70 (Suppl. 1), 127.

Sage, G. H. (1998). Sports participation as a builder of character? *The World and I*, 3, 629-641.

Spencer, H. (1949). *Education: intellectual, moral, and physical*. London: Watts.

Steinhaus, A. H. (1952). Principal principles of physical education. In *Proceedings of the College Physical Education Association*. Washington, DC: AAHPER, pp. 5-11.

Stoll, S. K. & Beller, J. M. (1998). *Sport as education: On the edge*. NY: Columbia University Teachers College.

Wilcox, R. C. (1991). Sport and national character: An empirical analysis. *Journal of Comparative Physical Education and Sport.*, XIII(1), 3-27.

Wren, D. A. (2005). *The history of management thought*. NJ: John Wiley & Sons.

Zeigler, E. F. (1972). A model for optimum professional development in a field called "X." In *Proceedings of the First*

Canadian Symposium on the Philosophy of Sport and Physical Activity. Ottawa, Canada: Sport Canada Directorate, pp. 16-28.

Zeigler, E. F. & Spaeth, M. J. (1975). *Administrative theory and practice in physical education and athletics*. Englewood Cliffs, NJ: Prentice-Hall.

Zeigler, E. F. (1976). In sport, as in all of life, man should be comprehensible to
man. *Journal of the Philosophy of Sport*, III, 121-126

Zeigler, E. F. (ed. & au.). (1994). *Physical education and kinesiology in North America: Professional and scholarly foundations.* Champaign, IL: Stipes.

Zeigler, E. F. (1995). *A selected, annotated bibliography of completed research on management theory and practice in physical education and athletics to 1972 (including a background essay).* Champaign, IL: Stipes.

Zeigler, E. F. (2003). Sport's plight in the postmodern world: Implications for the sport management profession," *International Journal of Sport Management*, 4(2), 93- 109.

Zeigler. E. F. (2005). *History and status of American physical education and educational sport.* Victoria, BC: Trafford.

PART 6
MAKING PERSONAL AND GROUP DECISIONS

All professionals, no matter in which field they are serving, are faced with decision-making day after day in their job situations. In the 1950s I discovered the Harvard Case Method Approach (i.e., *technique*, actually) to such decision-making used in business, one that had been developing for decades. Because it had not been used in our field previously, I subsequently wrote a text based on this approach titled *Administration of Physical Education and Athletics: The Case Method Approach* (Prentice-Hall, 1959). It had some success, but basically the field of physical education was "not ready" for it yet. I myself used the approach with considerable success in courses taught at The University of Michigan originally, and then subsequently at the University of Illinois from 1963 to 1971. Unfortunately the P-H editor wouldn't permit me to include information as to exactly how to use this approach in the text itself. He felt that doing that would be something contrary to the underlying rationale of the methodology. He insisted that there should be a *separate* instructor's manual. The end result was that many professors–prospective users of the approach–never saw the manual and simply "bumbled along" with a "common-sense approach."

I offer this information below here as something that can be useful to all professionals in their efforts to solve case problems in the ongoing endeavors. In addition to the slight modifications I made as they seemed advisable in my teaching, subsequently I also added information about how to carry out decision-making if it happened that there was an "ethical dimension" to the situation at hand requiring the making of a decision.

After the initial descriptive material below, a sample case analysis is included.

Next page, please...

DECISION-MAKING IN SPORT
AND PHYSICAL ACTIVITY EDUCATION
(WITH AN ETHICAL DIMENSION WHEN NEEDED)

Earle F. Zeigler, Ph.D.
The University of Western Ontario

The objective here is to provide the prospective sport and physical activity manager with information and a learning experience that will develop an understanding of a sound approach to decision-making. Such understanding (broadly speaking) includes:

(1) defining the problem or issue that should be resolved (*including whether one or more ethical issues is present*);

(2) considering the possible alternative courses of action;

(3) making a decision as to which alternative is best (everything considered);

(4) implementing the decision in the most effective and efficient manner possible; and

(5) evaluating the results of the decision after a reasonable period of time has elapsed.

Specifically, the approach recommended for daily use here is our adaptation based on long experience of what is generically called the Harvard case method (or technique) of decision-making.

All creatures on earth, human and non-human, have been making decisions since the evolutionary process began. A problem arose and a decision had to be made--e.g., fight, run, or hide. A choice was made according to certain alternatives that apparently were present in the problematic situation. As social life became increasingly complex, the decision-making process also became highly complicated as well. For example, what are the recommended steps that might be taken as an individual strives to make a rational decision? Also, what relationship do decisions have to the manager's value system? And where do (or should) emotions enter into the decision-making process? Further, can we establish a rough classification system for the various types of decisions (e.g., routine decisions), and under what conditions are decisions made (i.e., degree of risk)? Finally, what techniques have proven to be useful and valuable in the decision-making process?

As discussed earlier, an extensive body of literature on management theory and practice has developed since 1900. We explained further how management thought and theory has been characterized by steadily increasing complexity with the result that we now have what may be characteristically called a "management theory jungle." One of the several schools of thought that has been identified historically within this "morass" views management's primary function as decision-making, our topic in this present knowledge statement. If decision-making is so important, the manager's task is accordingly to gather as much information as possible about a subject and make decisions based on an analysis carried out with the best qualitative and quantitative techniques available. In essence, the latter of these two (quantitative techniques) is what was called operations research earlier before and during the World War II era and then titled "management science" more recently.

Research to this point has shown that human behavior in organizational settings manifests many similarities as one moves from educational institution, to retail store, to hospital, to welfare agency, or even to military unit. The evidence points to formal organizations exerting similar influence on the individuals functioning within their boundaries. The status hierarchy, for example, tends to cause dysfunctional effects wherever it appears. The resultant feelings emanating from satisfying and dissatisfying work are remarkably similar, also. Conflict between line and staff members of an organization erupts in the same manner, and this is especially true when subordinates have greater (or exclusive) knowledge and accompanying professional or technical efficiency than their hierarchical superiors. Admittedly, recent research suggests, and often recommends, newer types of organizational structures, but the bureaucratic organization and the types of individuals it "spawns," are still preponderantly operative.

If the above thought holds true, and the evidence points that way, it can be argued that organizations sponsoring sport, physical education, and physical recreation are influenced by the same confluence of organizational and psychological variables that prevail in the organizations cited above. This means that the decision-making process, and the manager's behavior as a decision-maker, function in similar "living organisms" where people pursue goals; seek personal identification; encounter opposition; react and (we hope) adjust to stress; strive to "stay alive" by adaptation, development of power, and growth.

The manager's role has typically been that of guiding and directing the resources of an organization from the input stage to the thruput stages and finally to output where objectives and goals may be achieved. Prior to decision-making at any stage of the process, the decision-maker must (1) receive information; (2) interpret and integrate it keeping many factors and influences well in mind; (3) consider alternative courses of action and make a rational choice; (4) execute the chosen course by appropriate action with the help of associates; and (5) evaluate along the way whether the implementation of the decision has resulted in effective and efficient action leading to positive results.

Managers in sport, physical activity education, and recreation settings are no different than any other managers in other settings. They too are continually faced with the making of decisions. The importance of making a correct decision is obvious; managers who make bad decisions usually suffer the consequences of their actions. (This is possibly more true if such decisions were made arbitrarily with no consultation.) Investigation and study have shown that the very large majority of managers in sport, physical education, and recreation settings are using intuition, judgment, and past experience to guide them in the decision-making process a great deal of the time. Inasmuch as a variety of highly useful models and tools are now readily available, but are not being used typically, this indicates a lack of understanding as to their possible effectiveness. It probably also indicates an inability to cope with them in a practical manner as well. To be fair to sport and physical education managers, it should be pointed out that managers in other fields are typically not using these tools and models very well or at all either. In fact, even among those who are presumably well versed in their use, they are often neglected because of lack of time, lack of applicability to a particular real-life situation, and the ever-present difficulty of quantifying all of the variables involved.

Some of the factors and influences that may affect organizational output throughout the implementation of the total management process are, for example, a lack of a clear set of explicitly stated, immediate objectives leading to the achievement of planned long range goals. Another factor influencing output might well be a degree of dysfunction arising from conflict between the formal and informal structure of an organization in a situation where workers are "out of touch" with the plans agreed to solely by the organization's managers. There may be a relationship here, also, between the leadership styles and personalities of the managers that negate open communication within the unit.

Years of involvement as a manager/administrator, as well as more than 30 years of experience with the case technique (of broader descriptive method) of teaching human relations and administration, led me to include a few thoughts here about the complexity of any administrative situation (Zeigler, 2010). This is so because of the large number of factors that may be involved in any case situation where decision-making is involved (e.g., past experience, one's present situation, economic incentive, personal attitude). The work situation itself and any changes that are occurring add to the mix. The group code within the organization, which in turn is affected by community standards and societal values and norms, are fundamental factors as well. Management says one thing, but management does another--this too can have an impact. In some circumstances certain factors indicated above could be the most important determinants of behavior; in others they might well be relatively insignificant. The task as you analyze a problem is, therefore, to gain as much perspective as possible. However, while responding to the facts, half-facts, and opinions as you see, hear, and assess them, you should keep in mind that each person views a situation differently. Such a realization in itself should often cause managers to hold back at least temporarily before initiating direct action to meet a problem.

Here we are discussing the achievement of at least elementary competency in decision-making through the use of a case method technique used extensively in law and medical training since the turn of the twentieth century. It is also true that the case method has been used as a teaching technique by business schools dating back to the 1920s. A notable example of this is the Harvard Business School in the United States and the subsequent complete adoption of this instructional approach by the University of Western Ontario School of Business Administration in Canada. Teachers in professional training programs know that the need to develop knowledge, competencies, and skills on the part of students in professional training programs is obvious and ever-present.

A common complaint of students in such programs in sport and physical education management or administration, however, is that adequate laboratory and/or field experiences are typically not available. And yet somehow this approach within professional preparation programs in physical education and athletics did not get introduced to the field until the late 1950s (Zeigler, 1959). Furthermore, oddly and interestingly, due mainly to several social influences (e.g., onrushing science and technology) and subsequent, prevailing educational essentialism, the case method technique of teaching human relations and administration is still used sparingly and sporadically in sport and physical education management.

Experience and past literature have shown that students react most favorably to this teaching technique because it promotes involvement and stimulates interest. Accordingly, because of the presumed need for a variety of teaching techniques in professional training, it is being recommended here for the burgeoning field of sport and physical activity management. This teaching method has such a great deal to offer that it deserves consideration for use more or less in all aspects of management training programs.

There is actually no fixed model, no infallible approach, or no standard pattern for the analysis of a case leading to improved decision-making. The tone of the analysis is important, because it is advisable that the manager avoid solutions that are primarily authoritarian if he or she wishes to improve human relations within the organization. The manager in assessing any problematic situation must develop as complete a mastery of the facts as possible, while keeping in mind that any case is characterized by facts, half-facts, and opinions. For this reason it imperative that a case be considered critically and that any opinions offered be weighed very carefully.

RECOMMENDED SEQUENTIAL STEPS IN THE DECISION-MAKING PROCESS

The manager should try to (Step No. 1) DETERMINE WHAT THE MAIN PROBLEM IS *AFTER* ENUMERATION OF THE VARIOUS SUB-PROBLEMS (Step No. 1). Formulating the best possible answers to the sub-issues or sub-questions helps to get to the heart of the analysis. A manager should strive to ascertain the exact question at issue, keeping in mind that it may be clear or obscured. Learning how to ask the right questions is basic to the art of administration.

> Note: If the main problem, or any of the sub-problem, is basically ethical in nature that should be noted and included in the analysis. An elementary three-step approach to ethical decision-making is included immediately below.

As can be readily appreciated, whether personal, professional, or environmental ethics are involved, the making of *ethical* decisions in no way resembles an exact science. Some might deplore such a situation, but in all probability the vast majority would find it desirable and wholesome. Nevertheless, the current dilemma faced by sport and physical activity managers in our society should be deplored--a situation where typically one hardly knows where to turn for some sound basis upon which to formulate an answer to just about any ethical problem that arises. What occurs, therefore, is that children and young adults are making choices, are forming value judgments, are experiencing emotions, and in a great many ways are acquiring an implicit view of life based on a "sense of life" (what Rand [1960, p. 31] called "a pre-conceptual equivalent of metaphysics, an emotional, subconsciously integrated appraisal of man and existence").

It is important, therefore, to help students approach ethical decision-making in as explicit a manner as possible. Such an approach should be one that could be useful to them throughout their adult lives. Yet such an approach should be one that they could possibly build upon throughout their lives as well. Over a period of time, with the advice of Professor Richard Fox of Cleveland State University, Ohio, U.S.A., a three-part plan of attack for ethical decision-making was devised. It was explained in considerable detail in E.F. Zeigler, *Applied Ethics for Sport and Physical Activity Managers,*. Bloomington, IN: Trafford, 2007. (It should be pointed out, however, that the instructor should make it very clear that this is only one approach with which they are being asked to experiment as they move toward greater sophistication in this vital aspect of their lives.) This plan of attack in its entirety includes the following three parts:

> Part A. Determine through the employment of a thee-step approach--from Kant to Mill to Aristotle--what the ethical or moral issue is in the specific case at hand. That is, proceed from a test of universalizability to A second test of (net) consequences, and finally to a third test of intentions.

> Part B. Once Part A has been carried out, proceed with Part B, or the layout of the argument (recommended as a jurisprudential argument in S. Toulmin. *The uses of argument.* NY: Cambridge University Press, 1964). In doing this, insert the universalizability maxim for Toulmin's warrant, the net consequences result of the presumably unethical action for the backing, and the intentions test items as possible conditions of exception or rebuttal.

> Part C. Thirdly, upon the completion of Parts A and B--if there is time and if human relations appear to have

166

played a significant part in the case problem--I have asked students to work their way through an even more detailed, overall approach (Part C) to ethical decision-making (as adapted from Manicas, P. T. and Kruger, A. N., *Essentials of logic.* NY: American Book Company, 1968 and Zeigler, E. F., *Decision-making in physical education and athletics administration: A case method approach.* Champaign, Il: Stipes Publishing Co., 1982). There are eight steps to this overall approach of Part C as follows:

(1) Determination of the main problem after consideration of the various sub-problems (including any with ethical implications).

(2) Explication of any knowledge-base, carry-forward information that may exist already in the mind of the student in connection with this sort of case problem (including ethical implications).

(3) Analysis of the main problem through application of a "three-step ethical approach" (the three tests listed above as recommended by Fox); this is integrated with a layout of the argument (based on Toulmin's approach).

(4) Analyze the various personalities and their relationships.

(5) Formulation of only those alternative solutions to the ethical problem that appear to be relevant, possible, and meaningful.

(6) Elaboration of the proposed alternative solutions involving the framing of warranted predictive statements (i.e., both pro's and con's).

(7) Selection of the preferred alternative solution (including initial tentative testing of the proposed solution prior to actual implementation--i.e., especially important if the case is actually a true one to be resolved).

(8) Assessment and determination of currently useful principles or generalizations for possible future use in similar situations.

(Note: These "principles" or "generalizations" should
supplement K-B,C-F principles suggested in "b"
above.)

Here you. as a management trainee, are being asked to read
the case carefully outside of class and then to draft an outline of a
case analysis using the headings listed immediately above (and
also followed in the sample case analysis below). Then you are to
carry out an actual case discussion with approximately five other
people in the class for approximately one class period (90 mins.
would be better if such an amount of time is available).

One member of the group of six should be selected to serve
as chairperson for the discussion. The chairperson should not
dominate the discussion or seek a predetermined goal. This
person would serve as (1) a resource person (if this were actually
the case), (2) an evaluator of progress, (3) an informed member of
the group, (4) a discussion chairperson, and (5) a summarizer.

The next recommended step (Step No. 2) we have named
KNOWLEDGE-BASE, CARRY-FORWARD GENERALIZATIONS,
admittedly a long, odd, and perhaps somewhat confusing
designation. All that this is, however, is an effort to determine
what is already known (the knowledge base) in regard to the
handling of similar problems or issues that may be "carried
forward" for use at present. That is, what principles or
generalizations can be brought for possible use to the case under
consideration at present?

(Note: Keep in mind that we are not for a minute
suggesting that there are basic principles of
administration that could apply here rigidly as
determinants of action to be taken in all case situations.
We are saying that there are currently useful
generalizations that may be carried forward for possible
use in similar situations. Obviously, there's a world of
difference between the former and the latter type of
information or knowledge.)

Step No. 3 involves a careful ANALYSIS OF THE VARIOUS
PERSONALITIES in the case and their relationships with each
other. In situations where human relations are involved--and they

are rarely not involved where qualitative decision-making comes into question--the interpersonal elements of a problematic situation can be vitally important.

At this juncture, brainstorming enters the picture, and it is time to FORMULATE POSSIBLE ALTERNATIVE COURSES OF ACTION--often as many as 10 or more (including variations). This is Step No. 4. Only plausible alternatives should be considered (i.e., that appear to be relevant, possible, and meaningful).

In Step No. 5, these alternatives for consideration should be "tested in advance," or elaborated upon, by the FRAMING OF WARRANTED PREDICTIVE STATEMENTS through the listing the pro's and con's of each, and then forecasting possible results if such-and-such an alternative were implemented as a solution (i.e., a decision to be taken).

In Step No. 6, the SELECTION OF THE PREFERRED ALTERNATIVE occurs (including initial tentative testing of the proposed solution prior to actual implementation).

> (Note: Despite all that has been written here, Lehrer (2009) warns us–in regard to the moral or ethical aspect of decision-making: "Our standard view of morality–the philosophical consensus for thousands of years–has been exactly backwards. We've assumed that our moral decisions are the by-products of rational thought…these arguments miss the central reality of *moral (my itals.)* decisions, which is that logic and legality have little to do with anything." See p. 171 of Lehrer's *How we decide* (Boston: Houghton Mifflin Harcourt, 2009). He claims that people have over the millennia become "inner-wired" and make such decisions emotionally and *then* seek to rationalize their decisions with rational thought.)

Next in line (Step No. 7) is the IMPLEMENTATION OF THE DECISION OR PLANNED COURSE OF ACTION as the preferred alternative to be carried out according to plan as to time, place, and method of execution.

EVALUATION OF THE RESULTS is Step No. 8 that should be carried out after a reasonable period of time has elapsed.

Next to last, in Step No. 9, any KNOWLEDGE, PRINCIPLES, OR CURRENTLY USEFUL GENERALIZATIONS gleaned from this experience should be added to the Knowledge Base Carry-Forward--possibly at the time the decision is implemented and then later revised (see Step No. 2 above) for possible future use in similar situations.

Note: In this case analysis provided as an example (MIDWESTERN UNIVERSITY A), you should understand that the results of implementing Step No. 8 could, of course, not be carried out until a period of time had elapsed.

Finally, to set the stage a bit further, in addition to the recommended steps to be followed in case analysis, we are offering below some hints to keep in mind as you carry out your own analysis. These might be called "traps to be avoided"....

1. Consider the "whole case" (i.e., don't jump to a rapid conclusion from inadequate data).
2. Don't always reason as the person who is the boss.
3. Don't always press for immediate action to be taken.
4. Don't memorize facts, conclusions, or principles from other cases.
5. Avoid solutions that are primarily authoritarian.
6. Don't be afraid to use your imagination, but weigh your opinions carefully.
7. Don't accept everything written or said as "gospel truth."
8. Don't make recommendations meaningless by over qualification; avoid phraseology with no meaning.
9. Don't regard each case as a wholly individual and isolated administrative involvement.
10. Don't develop a case of "retrospective should-itis" (i.e., he should have done that; she should have done this; they must do that. In other words, be prospective! The case tells what happened; now "where do we go from

here?" How can the administrative process be improved?

11. Don't re-hash too much of the case as written in your analysis.
12. Keep the "tone" of your analysis constructive.
13. Avoid "either-or" thinking based on the invoking of immutable principles.

Note: The author first became involved with this approach to teaching human relations more than 60 years ago. Some of the above suggestions have been adapted initially from M.P. McNair and H.L. Hansen (1949). *Problems in marketing.* NY: McGraw-Hill, pp. 22-25.

Finally, I urge you to keep firmly in mind that the objective of this method of analysis is to help you as a manager to develop POWER by providing an opportunity to think in a constructive, orderly manner when facing new problematic situations. When you, as manager, finally do propose a solution, try to make recommendations that will improve the management process for the future. Through this type of analysis you will develop your powers of discrimination and generalization.

APPENDIX:
A SAMPLE CASE: MIDWESTERN UNIVERSITY A

Earle F. Zeigler, The Univ. of Western Ontario
Robert L. Case, Sam Houston State University
Steve Timewell, The Univ. of Western Ontario

Note: This sample case, (MIDWESTERN UNIVERSITY A), was an actual situation that occurred with names and places disguised. A detailed analysis of this case is offered immediately below for your POSSIBLE use. It is designed to provide an experience in the application of the case method technique to problem-solving and decision-making in sport and physical activity education. Remember that the objective of this method of analysis leading to the making of a decision is to help you as a manager develop power by providing an opportunity to think in a constructive, orderly manner when facing new, problematic situations. Through this type of analysis you will develop your powers of discrimination and generalization. When you finally do make a decision and propose a solution, do your best to make recommendations that will improve the management process for the future.

This particular case and analysis also included a consideration of possible ethical implications. However, since this approach to the case method technique of decision-making in sport and physical activity management can be used very well without *detailed* consideration being given to the ethical aspects of any given case, we decided to leave that step out of this presentation initially so that it all wouldn't seem too complex. A brief section offering an elementary three-step approach to ethical decision-making will be included at the end of the case analysis below.

> Note: Williams Sanders is an instructor working on his doctoral degree at Midwestern University. On February 1, 1995, he sent the following letter to Prof. T.C. Collins, Chairperson, Department of Sport and Physical Education, Midwestern University:

Dear Dr. Collins:

As you know, Head Coach Courtney and I have just completed the teaching of PE 156 (Wrestling), a course that we have handled jointly for the past few years. This year I had developed a new grading scheme that we presented to the students at the first class period. We agreed that I would determine the written work to be completed, and the skills we were to teach were those that Coach Tom stresses typically.

Both of us graded students at various times during the semester on their ability at the skills. Tom asked me, as usual, to grade all of the written work. This I did, and all grades, including attendance, were listed on a large chart kept in Mr. Courtney's office. (Near the end of the term, incidentally, a number of the students were complaining to both Tom and me that he [Tom] had been marking them absent incorrectly.)

While grading the written work, I noticed that one student, a prominent Midwestern athlete, turned in someone else's class notebook (a regularly assigned project) under his own name. I actually remembered grading this particular notebook over Xmas vacation a year ago. He also handed in several other assignments at this time, ones that were actually due at the middle of the semester. He explained that injury during the fall season had prevented him from getting them in on time. Unfortunately, this was not his own work either. I notified Coach Courtney immediately since he is, of course, technically my superior with professorial status. He suggested that I give him the papers and the notebook, and that he himself would confront the student and his coach together.

The following day Coach Tom informed me that, despite the young man's plagiarism, Courtney and Slaughter (the student's coach) agreed that the athlete should re-work his notebook and assigned papers. As punishment he would be asked to complete an extra assignment recommended by me. In this way his failing grade could be raised sufficiently so as not to make it impossible for him to get off academic probation. The student came to see me; received the extra assignment; and was to return everything to me when it was completed. Then I would change the grade if his work merited such revision.

My complaint is that I never saw the results. I asked Coach Tom about it, and he explained that he had received the work, graded it, and had misplaced it at home. I decided to check out the grade submitted and learned that this person, and many other varsity athletes, received a grade of A in the course, while others more deserving received B's and C's. Regretfully, I must charge Coach Tom with dishonesty and a lack of professional ethics.

Very sincerely yours,
William Sanders, Asst. Coach

ANALYSIS OF CASE
(Including Ethical Implications)

1. Sub-Problems (leading to determination of the Main Problem):

    a. The seemingly evident plagiarism of the athlete--ethically wrong.

    b. Courtney, despite pre-determined grading agreement with Sanders that the latter would grade written work, grades Sanders' written work himself and doesn't even allow Sanders to see the submission--ethically wrong.

    c. Athlete evidently was using his "athletic profile" for a special privilege (i.e., to be able to get away with handing assignment in late)--ethically wrong.

    d. The fact that upon examination Sanders discovered that various varsity athletes received A's in the course, while others that Sanders felt actually did better re- only B's and C's--ethically wrong.

    e. The fact that Courtney initially went to the athlete's coach to discussed the athlete's predicament (a person who was already on academic probation) and seemingly took his plagiarism so casually; one wonders whether they (Courtney and Slaughter) ever even intended that he should complete his work for the course--ethically wrong.

    f. The very fact that Coach Courtney showed truly unfair advantage to a varsity athlete, allowing him to escape any punishment for an offense that some other student might be severely punished for, or even dismissed from the university--ethically wrong.

    g. Sanders may have erred by accepting the "substitute

174

plan" recommended by Courtney after the initial plagiarism had been detected and reported by Sanders to Courtney.

After extensive discussion, the MAIN ETHICAL PROBLEM was determined to be Sub-problem #f above (Courtney's Ethical Conduct)

2. Knowledge Base Carry-Forward
   (Principles or Generalizations generally accepted)

   a. Plagiarism is cheating, an unacceptable practice in higher education.
   b. Unless there are truly extenuating circumstances, we must live up to commitments we agree upon with others.
   c. Granting "special" privileges to some people and not to their peers is unfair and will create serious problems.
   d. Athletics is but one of many aspects of university life, and should be kept in proper perspective with the overall educational function of higher education.

3. Employment of the Three-Step Approach Related to Ethics

   a. Universalizability or Consistency (Test #1)

      Based on society's values and norms, and that universities are regarded as pattern-maintenance organizations where honesty and integrity are absolutely essential, proven plagiarism is most serious

   b. (Net) Consequences (Test #2)

      Proven dishonesty by teachers and coaches that is somehow not punished could seriously damage the university's reputation and place the institution's future in jeopardy

   c. Intentions (Test #3)

      The voluntary and/or involuntary nature of Coach

175

Courtney's actions must be ascertained, and then appropriate action should be taken based on the findings (e.g., dismissal for cause)

4. Integration of Triple-Play Approach with Argument Layout

Data	So, (necessarily)	Conclusion

Head Wrestling Coach Courtney is reported by his teaching assistant as having shown extreme favoritism to a tendered athlete from another sport, a man who is on academic probation and who has evidently committed plagiarism

The department head should make every effort to learn the true facts of the situation, and then should take appropriate action based on his findings (e.g., dismissal for cause)

Since
Warrant

Unless
Rebuttal or Exception

Based on society's values and norms, and that universities are regarded as pattern-maintenance organizations where honesty and integrity are absolutely essential, an offense such as proven plagiarism is most serious

It turns out that Courtney actually did forget and did grade the manual himself which was excellent in all regards

Universalizability (Test 1)

and/or

Because
Backing

Courtney was under some external pressure; felt that he simply had no recourse other than to provide help for the athlete who was on academic probation

Proven dishonesty by teachers and coaches that is somehow not punished could seriously damage a university's reputation and place the institution's future in jeopardy

and/or

Consequences (Test 2)

Courtney was old, near retirement, had an excellent record otherwise, offered an apology; corrected the well-intentioned error; thus, clemency was felt to be in order

176

and/or

It turned out that the
whole problem has been
greatly exaggerated by
Sanders who had it in for
Courtney and perhaps hoped
to succeed to the position
if Courtney were dismissed

Intentions (Test 3)

Key: Argument Layout (Toulmin, 1964)

D = data (a statement of a situation that prevails,
     including evidence, elements, sources, samples of facts)
C = conclusion (claim or conclusion that we are seeking to
     establish)
W = warrant (practical standards or canons of argument
     designed to provide an answer to the question. "How do
     you get there?")
Q = modal qualifier (adverbs employed to qualify con-
     clusions based on strengths of warrants--e.g., neces-
     sarily, probably)
R = conditions of exception (conditions of rebuttal or
     exception that tend to refute the conclusion)
B = backing (categorical statements of fact that lend
     further support to the 'bridge-like" warrants)

5. Personalities and Ethical Relationships:

   a. There appears to be a difference in the way which the
      coaches at Midwestern University regard academic work
      and offenses and infractions that might occur. Courtney
      evidently felt it was more important for a top athlete to
      be eligible than to be honest, as did Slaughter--but
      Sanders didn't agree.
   b. At least some athletes at Midwestern figured you could
      get away with handing in someone else's work--or else

177

this one wouldn't have tried it. If this is true, this could affect a professional program most seriously.

    c. Even if everything that Courtney said was true (e.g., he had found it to be worth an A grade), what about the other varsity athletes who Sanders felt was receiving grades that were to high (relatively speaking, that is).

    d. If Courtney had been under some external pressure to see to it that the athlete became eligible again, one would think that Sanders might be aware of this--but perhaps not.

6. Relevant Alternatives Open to One of the Participants:

> Note: We have chosen to view the matter from the standpoint of Wm. Sanders, Asst. Coach)

7. Preferred Alternative Solution (Confront Courtney before reporting him to departmental chairperson)

+++

Are We Deluding Ourselves?

According to Jonah Lehrer and his work in neuroscience (!), humans have been deluding themselves if they think use logic to determine their responses to ethical problems that arise in the course of their daily lives. Neuroscience, he claims, is telling us that moral judgment is like aesthetic judgment. In other words, Kant was wrong! The "rational brain" does not analyze the problematic situation "scientifically"! What we do, Lehrer says, is to react emotionally to the situation, and THEN we reason our way to some sort of justification for the way we feel! If this is so, Lehrer has "thrown a large monkey wrench" into the question of ethical decision-making". (See J. Lehrer's How We DECIDE, Boston, MA: Houghton Mifflin Harcourt, 2009)
+++

a. Initially, Sanders should have taken a stand against Courtney when he first learned how the matter was to be handled. Perhaps he should have done so . . . .

Pro--maybe he could have convinced Courtney to quickly retrace his steps and change what he had just done (i.e., submit a false grade, etc.).
Con--Courtney might have been angry at being challenged and would have attempted to somehow "cover his tracks".

b. After Sanders discovered the plagiarism, he should have quietly referred it to Collins and not become so openly involved.

Pro--by "playing it safe" his position might be more secure.
Con--his conscience might have bothered him because somehow in North American culture a "sneaky Judas" is especially condemned when an action becomes generally known.

c. Before taking any action (i.e., writing the letter), Sanders should have confronted Coach Courtney about this matter; he should also ask him to justify the especially high grades for all the tendered athletes (with lower grades for others); this would be somewhat more ethical than "going over his head" immediately.

See pro's and con's in Question #6 below (Preferred Alternative Solution).

d. Sanders could have contacted Coach Slaughter to discuss the situation. Slaughter's reaction might have provided addiional evidence (one way or the other).

Pro--this would have to be handled most carefully. It could have caused him to get back to Courtney rapidly to call the whole affair off. It would also give Sanders a stronger case either way it turned out.
Con--Sanders would be "sticking his neck out" even further and this might cause a violent reaction from the authorities in the Athletic Association directed at injuring

Sanders' job standing and his future.

e. Sanders could check grades over the most recent years to see
if there had been a pattern indicating that athletes were
being treated in a special manner.

Pro--this might also strengthen Sanders' case or
it might dissuade him from writing the letter if
nothing seemed to have been wrong. It could also have
been used in connection with #c above to try to convince
Courtney of the error of his actions.
Con--it might be difficult to get the former grade
books without arousing suspicion on Courtney's part.

f. Once the complaint has been filed, Sanders should leave the
matter at that and remove himself as far as possible from having
anything to do with it (ethical?).

Pro--one is tempted to do this if possible, and it
does leave the accuser somewhat less tainted by the
whole affair.
Con--this possibility rarely develops, mainly because
the accuser is need as a witness and thereby is forced
to take a stand.

g. Sanders should somehow get the information to Dr. Collins
anonymously; in this way he might conceivably escape from any
responsibility in the matter.

Pro--this could really be playing it safe, and it
might work.
Con--Sanders' conscience would probably have bothered
him, and also receipt of such an anonymous
accusation might well be ignored.

6&7. Preferred Alternative Solution (Confront Courtney before
        reporting him to departmental chairperson)

Alternative #c above:

Before taking any action (i.e., writing the letter), Sanders should have confronted Coach Courtney about this matter; he should also ask him to justify the especially high grades for all the tendered athletes (with lower grades for others); this would be somewhat more ethical than "going over his head" immediately.

Pro's	Con's
Would have gone through proper channels	- By confronting Courtney there might have been some "backlash"
- Courtney would have known that Sanders was aware of his unfair practices and might be reporting him to the administrator	- Improper grading might have led to punishment of Courtney and his possible dismissal anyhow
- Sanders would have given Courtney a chance to explain what he had been doing by offering some rationale for it	- If Courtney could not have ex plained his actions, he would be working mightily to harm Sanders and have him "black-balled by the Athletic Assoc.
- If Sanders could have convinced Courtney that his grading practices were then maybe something might have been worked out before the chairman was notified	- If an investigation had taken place-and Courtney some-how was innocent- ridiculous, Sanders would have been in a most precarious position to to say the least

8. Currently Useful Principles or Generalizations

> Note: These are recommended as a result of the case analysis, being added to the Knowledge Base Carry-forward in #2 above.

a. Keep in mind that there is a considerable range of opinion in this culture as to how ethical conduct is perceived.
b. It is most important that teachers/coaches set high ethical standards for themselves.
c. Every effort should be made to keep the lines of communication open with colleagues in a work situation.
d. When team teaching is being carried out, it is especially important to have the policies and procedures to be used spelled out most carefully in advance of the actual teaching situation.

PART 7
A MARKETING ORIENTATION FOR
AN ATHLETIC/RECREATION PROGRAM

(Co-author John T. Campbell, M.A.,
Toronto, ON, Canada)

Introduction

All North American enterprises faced what has been called a "quality imperative" in the final quarter of the 20th century. The same idea is still paramount today in the face of a recession coupled with increasing global competition. Doing business is simply radically different from the past when customers could be taken for granted. In a global marketplace where quality is the watchword of competition, business needs to rededicate itself to excellence by world standards..

Similarly, all administrators/managers of athletic/physical recreation programs were forced to consider a revised marketing orientation, a whole new set of postulates for them to accept or reject. Competitive athletics and physical recreation and intramurals--all recreation for that matter--have typically been regarded as extra-curricular. A small percentage of people would be willing to accord them co-curricular status. Moreover, an even smaller percentage would accord them curricular status *if* certain conditions prevailed. We fall into this latter category.

Accordingly, our belief does not rest with those who believe that so-called educational athletics and physical recreation should be confined almost completely to club sports, perhaps under the intramurals program, with a separate structure for intercollegiate football and basketball (and any other sport that pays for itself through gate receipts). Nor does it rest with those at the other extreme who argue that the main problem is simply that of "learning to market the product better," thereby creating sufficient profit to meet all demands.

We do believe fully in the "quality imperative," in "striving for excellence" in any activity considered acceptable in the educational environment. This means promoting it to the extent that such striving is compatible with high educational standards (such standards admittedly being difficult to define). Hence, to lay the philosophical groundwork for the first section of this chapter, we are in favor of scholarships for athletes who are striving for excellence, *but only where they have proven financial need*! This is just the same as we are in favor of financial aid for *any bona fide* student with talent in one of a number of recognized "cultural talents"--*where there is proven need*! Our assumption is that worthy, needy students must have sufficient time to devote to the full development of their talents.

Because competitive sport, for example, has only rarely received full educational status at any educational level, full support of athletic programs has been an ever-present budgetary problem. Further, with rare exceptions, gate receipts are *always* of concern, a situation that has often placed great pressure on athletic directors and head coaches of certain revenue sports to produce winning teams. This fact has resulted in a multitude of human and material problems far too numerous to list here. These problems are well known by all, and it would serve no purpose to dwell on any of them at this point.

In the final quarter of the 20th century, at least two factors exacerbated this continuing problem: the financial plight of higher education in general, and the Title IX issue specifically (where increased allotments were mandated for women's competitive sport to achieve a semblance of "equal opportunity"). In addition, a third problem caused concern for all facets of the economy: Those of us related to sport and recreation were victimized by those social forces as well--economic inflation, mini-depressions, and the occasional period of what has become known as "stagflation" (the stagnant economy accompanied by inflation in the 1980s). We began to get the uneasy feeling that college athletics, as we have known it, might eventually be forced to price itself out of the market. As Bole indicated in 1970, alternative methods of financing athletics should be explored before the situation becomes impossible (p. 93). It would indeed be a tragedy if we end up with truncated programs made up of intercollegiate football and basketball only. Under such conditions, all other competitive sports with certain exceptions (e.g., wrestling at Lehigh, hockey at Michigan) would be relegated to minor sport status and would have to follow the extramural or club sport pattern (not to denigrate these activities, of course).

Further, to a greater or lesser extent, the financial outlay for athletic scholarships has hung around the necks of United States athletic directors, especially, like the fabled albatross for many decades. Then, an action that is now history occurred, many state legislatures because of federal Title IX legislation were rightfully required to appropriate funds for athletic scholarships for women as well. Under certain conditions, as mentioned above, we are not questioning this practice for either sex, but the fact cannot be escaped that a tremendous burden has been placed on athletic budgets. This is obviously one more consideration that must evidently be placed into the athletics "planning mix" on a continuing basis.

The question of athletic scholarships has in the 21st century moved--seemingly almost inevitably--to the forefront in Canada as well. Starting in the 1950s the subject of improvement of national and international sport became a political issue. As governments turned over, there were pressures on the new government to bring competitive sport to parity at least with countries of similar wealth and population. The federal government in Canada did institute so-called, third-party scholarships for "carded athletes" with national standing some years ago. This caused some problems, but by and large this *nondirective* approach (insofar as the universities were concerned) did not cause as many problems as had been anticipated by those who were in opposition to the move. Then some of the provincial government entered the picture similarly (e.g., British Columbia), with both levels of government using lottery receipts to help offset the added financial burden. Some universities in the east and mid–west also began to grant certain financial aid even before the regulations were relaxed. The result in the 1990s was two levels of university competition--one for those who grant athletic scholarships, and one for those who don't (not mentioning the few "under-the-table" institutions. What the future holds is anybody's guess, but we can only hope that academic standards will not be lowered, and that extensive programs of competitive sport for men and women will not have to be curtailed because of continuing inflation and declining income (the latter being derived almost completely from student fees and--more recently--from certain provincial aid programs).

In the United States especially, athletic departments have necessarily felt that they should do all in their power--presumably within the letter and the spirit of the rules within higher education--to produce winning teams. This has been particularly true for those sports that have produced significant amounts of revenue in the past, money that has literally supported teams in other sports where gate receipts were light or nonexistent.

Background of the Marketing Orientation Concept

The time is now long past when a chairperson or director should have given consideration to his or her institution's stance in regard to what is now known as the *marketing concept*. This business phenomenon began in the 1940s and 1950s and has served business and industry and a number of athletic departments so well ever since. The question is whether the many social changes since have created a social climate that requires a whole new set of postulates for the administrator/manager no matter what the size or scope of the sport or physical recreation enterprise. The basic question to be faced, of course, is whether the "Canham marketing philosophy" (the former AD of Michigan at Ann Arbor) can work for all colleges and universities--or whether it is unique for certain universities in specific geographic regions only. To understand this problem more fully, it is necessary first to review briefly the development of the marketing concept since its origination.

Marketing is typically defined as activities that accelerate the movement of goods or services from the manufacturer to the consumer. Thus, it is marketing whether one is talking about advertising, distribution, merchandising, product-planning, promotion, publicity, and even transportation and warehousing. Phrased in a slightly different way, marketing involves the performance of "business activities" that influence the flow of goods and services from the producer to the consumer or user. Certain activities take place before the marketing process sets in (i.e., the identification of marketing needs, desires, and preferences). In other words, the market needs develop, and then typically a business organization is developed to meet those demands.

The development of the marketing concept can be characterized as a response from business to a society that was steadily acquiring more buying power. The personal income of the average family rose steadily so that life's basic essentials used up a smaller proportion of a person's salary. The nature of the consumer's demands changed along with the rising production levels. Then, as the average person's discretionary income increased further, there was a dramatic rise in the demand for services in the final quarter of the 20th century. Concurrently, we witnessed a multitude of technologic innovations with many new variations of distribution patterns.

As the social environment gradually altered, and a different lifestyle emerged for many families, the business community was affected as well. Unions demanded shorter workweeks, but in time the pressure of continuing inflation gradually forced both parents in a family to seek work. This pressure, coupled with increasing freedom enabling women to escape (to a degree) from being homebound almost completely, has resulted in a situation at the beginning of the 21st century where two-thirds of married women are gainfully employed. All of this caused increased demands for commercial recreation, labor-saving devices in the home, opportunities for travel, and opportunities for in-service education.

The result of this societal "upheaval" was a variety of demands for what might be called heterogeneity of goods and services that soon brought about the introduction of the concept of "market segmentation." Each segment had its own discrete desires, needs, and preferences. Thus, businesses found it mandatory to develop and maintain a market-strategy plan. When a company determined which its preferred segment of the market was, decisions could then be made sensibly about which directions should be taken with product development, pricing, distribution, and communication.

Here it is important to distinguish between the concepts of "market segmentation" and "product differentiation." The latter term relates to the different brands of a product *as viewed by* the prospective consumer. Here we are, for example, seeking a better understanding of the marketing orientation for competitive athletics. In this connection, this idea of product differentiation may be one way for athletics to appeal to its presumed market segment. By that we mean that competitive athletics in *educational* institutions can, and probably should be, offered to that segment of the population interested in it on the basis of the *unique* qualities that only it possesses. It may take market research of a social–psychology nature to figure this out scientifically, but it would be worth the time and effort to discover the answers to this important question.

Marketing Management for Athletics & Physical Recreation

Everything stated to this point may be regarded as history. In addition, I admit the difficulty of gaining true historical perspective on the immediate past. However, present demands are confronting us squarely with a *quality imperative*. Hence, I will now offer some suggestions and recommendations that may be helpful as directors of athletics prepare to face the evolving internal and external environments of the 21st century. As we think of the total process of sport marketing (see Figure 1 below), keep in mind that there can be three categories of parameters and/or variables that influence the entire undertaking as follows: (1) environmental *non–controllable* parameters (constraints or opportunities); (2) internal *controllable* variables; and (3) *partially controllable* variables (that may be external or internal). It is important that all concerned--athletic directors, sport managers, business managers, governing boards, etc.--understand how strong these factors may be.

The environmental *non-controllable* parameters may be viewed as external influences that must be considered seriously. They are such persistent historical problems as: (1) the influence

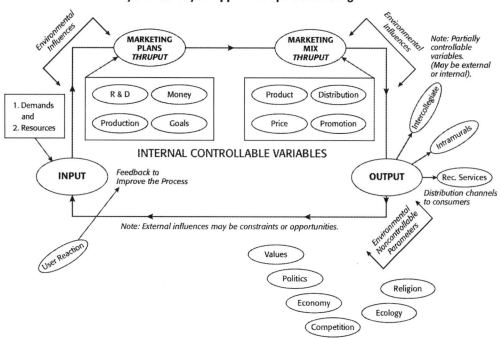

FIGURE 1

Systems Analysis Applied to Sport Marketing

of the society's values and norms; (2) the influence of politics (or the type of political state in which the organization is functioning); (3) the influence of economics (or the type and state of the economy); (4) the influence of religion; (5) the influence of ecology; and (6) the presence of competition (see bottom right of Figure 1 above). Not designated here, but often extremely powerful, is the influence of nationalism in one of several forms.

Initially, the business organization perceives certain societal demands and/or needs. Depending on the specific circumstances, the society and/or the organization's backer respond by making available (initially or potentially) material and human resources such as available capital, some level of market position or reputation, and a management team of good, bad, or indifferent stature. Of course, all of this is ultimately part of the total management process itself. After the initial *input* stage has been started, we are really describing functions that occur within the larger management process that is typically characterized by such terms as planning, organizing, staffing, directing, and controlling.

What we are actually presenting here is a model of a systems approach to sport marketing. Marketing plans include such factors or elements as (1) the guidance of stated objectives or goals; (2) the infusion of monetary resources; (3) the availability of a production unit; and (4) the services of a research and development division. This is the first stage of the *thruput* phase of a systems approach and also the first set of *internal controllable variables*. If we relate a business model to sport marketing, however, it becomes obvious immediately that all of these factors have typically not been available to the manager of athletics in as sophisticated a form as they might be or should be (e.g., a research and development division).

As we move forward to the second stage of the *thruput* phase of this systems approach--the stage in which the marketing mix is developed--it is readily apparent that the administrator/manager is confronted with four major elements which are the same ones that must be considered in any business. They are (1) the product presented to the public; (2) the price charged for that product; (3) the ways the product will be distributed to the public (i.e., the athletics competition, the fitness club services, etc.); and (4) the means employed to promote the product. We can readily understand how the proportions of the marketing mix may necessarily change in order to produce the most profitable marketing mix. For example, an administrator could soon be priced out of the market by charging too much for tickets, or by charging the budget too heavily for advertising within the total promotional effort.

The *output* stage of our systems approach correlates with the distribution channels of a marketing system. These channels--which in connection with sport marketing are usually intercollegiate (or interscholastic) athletics, intramural sports and sport clubs, and recreational sports and developmental physical activity services, are designated as *output*. They may also be regarded as *partially controllable variables*. This variability is present because–in the final analysis–the athletics director or manager is confronted with output variables that he or she only partially controls.

Finally, then, we have arrived at the user or consumer stage of our systems approach. It is this point that the administrator soon discovers whether the distribution channels of his/her presumably educational business--whether public, semi-public, or private--are functioning poorly, adequately, or in superior fashion. Here we think initially of success from a profit-and-loss standpoint. However, in the control phase of the management process, it is absolutely imperative that the manager obtain various types of feedback from consumers as to their satisfaction with the entire process. This means that the administrator should measure and then evaluate the several products regularly and systematically (i.e., determine how the three channels of distribution (or program offerings are being received by the various consumer levels). In the case of a college or university, for example, these consumers would be the students, faculty, staff, alumni, higher administration, board of trustees or governors, and the general public. Further, at all points during the entire process, the sport and physical activity program--in total or in part--may encounter favorable, neutral, or unfavorable influences from the many external non–controllable parameters (e.g., state of the economy, competition, poor weather).

Concluding Statement

From many conversations with others who are also involved with the program management, and based on a careful analysis of the literature, we believe that few athletics and physical activity managers have ever had (or taken) the opportunity to invoke a systems concept that could help them to understand fully how such an involved process are (1) market planning, (2) the development of a marketing mix, (3) the careful arrangement of the distribution channels, and (4) the feedback from the users, could work in its entirety. Of course, we have all been involved in the various phases of our positions in a piecemeal fashion. However, unless the manager came to the position with a background in theory, he presumably did not have the knowledge and competencies to envision the entire process in the light of operations research. As stated above, who ever heard of a research and development unit for an intercollegiate athletic program before the time when such educational institutions found themselves running "business enterprises."

What should we do specifically to provide sufficient (potential) customer orientation with our several programs? How can we move ahead to meet the immediate demands of a North American *quality imperative*? The answer would seem to be that all of us should have an introduction to what might be called *strategic market planning* in which we learn specifically what steps must be taken to develop a sound, realizable plan for our respective organizations. Then, once we have achieved an overall conceptualization of the entire subject, each of us will be in a position to study the skeleton, theoretic *evaluation schedule* offered below in this chapter.

> (Note: As it happened this "theoretic model" was actually adapted to a real life situation in the Physical Recreation & Intramurals Program of The University of Western Ontario.

Proceeding from this point, the reader would be ready to adapt the evaluation schedule to his or her own needs in arriving at a decision as to long range aims and immediate objectives. From this assessment, the reader (as a prospective or present administrator/manager) can build an effective strategic marketing plan that will result in a customer-oriented program involving more than (1) an expression of good intentions, (2) a variety of promotional tricks, and (3) a program of good, bad, or indifferent quality. This will be difficult, especially at a time when it is urgent also that academic subject-matter be taught more effectively. However, it must be done because physical activity education & recreation are important in the education of all young people. As a manager, you may indeed respond that you already have a marketing plan in place. If this is true, that's fine. However, you may then wish to employ this Evaluation Schedule by adapting it to mesh with (or enhance) your present plan. There is always room for improvement as we strive for excellence in an ever more competitive environment.

Appendix
Program Evaluation Schedule
(Based on Strategic Market Planning)

The growing importance of the marketing concept as an aid to the development of sport, fitness, and recreation programs in the various aspects of our society led to the development of an evaluation schedule. This schedule is designed for use by an individual, a group of individuals, or other interested parties to evaluate the present status of an organization's marketing plan (including the marketing mix). Strategic market planning, as envisioned here, consists of five steps or stages as follows: (1) Definition of the organization, (2) Status of the organization (including present budget and resource allocation), (3) Evaluation of the present marketing plan, (4) Assessment of the present marketing mix, and (5) Determination of the future marketing plan (including a new marketing mix and subsequent budgetary implications).

At each stage of this evaluation or assessment, those concerned are asked to check off their reactions in regard to (1) general administration and (2) various aspects of their programs, thereby possibly detecting problem areas. (An individual rating omitted or added would change the divisor accordingly [up or down] in each step.) In addition to the evaluation of status, the schedule may also be used as an aid in setting up a marketing plan for the future.

The schedule is primarily a self-rating device for use by those in a position to respond *knowledgeably* to the questions asked. These queries have to do with facilities, personnel, program, and services. The overall program (and/or individual subunits or subdivisions ratings) provide both individual and/or group analyses depending on how the instrument is used. It will help determine whether any changes are required in the operation of your present marketing plan. The schedule proceeds sequentially through the five steps of strategic market planning as outlined above.

The schedule may be used with a numerical scoring system. Scoring for each item (i.e., Excellent = 5, Very Good = 4, etc.) is from the highest rating to the lowest. The adjectives or numbers you assign should correspond to the present effectiveness of that aspect of the organization or its subunits under consideration.

Instructions for Using the Evaluation

Since the evaluation schedule is a self-rating device, the director or chairperson, as manager, leader, and coordinator of the overall management team in the organization, may wish to have the different people holding a variety of duties and responsibilities fill out a checklist. Although he and the unit heads may wish to apply different weightings to the various sets of responses that are received, this is nevertheless a good way to receive a number of opinions on the success, mediocrity, or failure of the present (marketing) plan of operation being employed.

Each item should be rated separately. At the end of each STEP (of the total of five) is a space for the mathematical average of all items in that phase to be figured. Later these averages can be transferred to the summary section at the end. From this summary total, an overall average can be determined by simple arithmetic. The qualitative and numerical ratings are as follows:

    EX---excellent.........................5
    VG---very good......................4
    AC---acceptable...................3
    FA---fair..................................2
    PO---poor.............................1

Notes:

(1) The evaluation schedule has been set up with the Physical Recreation and Intramurals of one university of mind. *With a minimum of changes throughout the schedule, it may be very easily adapted to any program desired (i.e., college, university, commercial organization, non-profit agency, governmental agency, etc.)*

(2) Ratings of individual items may be averaged where and when this is desired. This point should be kept in mind since averaged ratings of all individuals items lumped together tend to move the overall averaged scores toward the midpoint of 2.5

(Please proceed to STEP ONE below)

STEP ONE: DEFINITION OF THE ORGANIZATION

Please indicate how well these statements reflect your personal beliefs and opinions

Numerical
Score
(e.g., VG = 4)

A. PURPOSE (or overall program definition)

1. The Physical Recreation and Intramurals Program at The University of Western Ontario should be one of four programs within the Faculty of Kinesiology.

   _____

2. PRIP should be supported by student activity fees, non-student membership fees, charges for special services, and, to a limited extent, by general university funding.

   _____

3. It should maintain its administrative office in the University Community Centre with the Sports and Recreation Services Office in Thames Hall.

   _____

4. The mission of PRIP should be to motivate members of the university community to be responsible for their own health and fitness, and to promote and facilitate their

involvement in wholesome physical activity
to carry out this responsibility. _____

5. To do this PRIP should offer a balanced
program of wholesome activities that involve
learning and practicing sport, physical
fitness, and recreational skills in various
settings ranging from casual to highly
structured. _____

6. PRIP's activities should be divided into
the following units: (1) drop-in (casual)
activities; (2) non-credit instruction; (3)
intramural competitive sports; (4) physical
fitness; (5) aquatics; (6) sport clubs. _____

B. PRODUCT AND MARKET SCOPE
(from an overall standpoint)

1. Generally, how well have the target
markets (i.e. clients) been defined
within the University Community? _____

2. Generally, have the services provided
been sufficiently differentiated to meet
the clients' needs? _____

3. Has market segmentation been sufficiently achieved (i.e., by separating
the market into categories and thereby developing an adequate market
profile)? _____

3.1 Who? Do we adequately understand whom we are dealing with
in each category? _____

3.2 Where? Are we serving clients
in the place where they want to
be served? _____

3.3 <u>When</u>? Are we serving clients when they want to be served?

           _____

3.4 <u>How Many</u>? Are we serving a sufficient number of clients in the program offering with which they want to be involved?

           _____

3.5 <u>How</u>? Are we serving clients in the way they wish to be served (i.e., quality of service or instruction?

           _____

3.6 <u>Type of Client</u>? Are we reaching those clients who need to be served?

           _____

C. AVERAGE RATING— ORGANIZATIONAL DEFINITION =

           _____

<u>Note</u>: Please add up the NUMERICAL ratings the column above. Then divide the total by the <u>number</u> (DIVISOR) of ratings you felt qualified or able to make. For example, if you felt that you could answer 10 of the 14 questions, 5 of them with a rating of 3 and 5 with a rating of 4, your total would be 35. 35 divided by 10 = 3.5. Thus, you have evaluated the ORGANIZATIONAL DEFINITION of the PRIP with a 3.5 (or in the middle between Very Good [VG] and Acceptable [AC]).

<u>STEP TWO: STATUS OF THE ORGANIZATION</u>

<u>Note</u>: Be careful here to evaluate A here from the standpoint of your involvement with a <u>specific</u> unit (e.g., Fitness) and C based on your evaluation of the <u>overall</u> Program.

<u>Numerical</u>
<u>Score</u>
(e.g., AC = 3)

A. MARKET OPPORTUNITIES
(assessing your unit
<u>specifically</u>)   _____

1. Market Share:

   1.1 <u>Current</u>? Is my unit (interest
       area) serving the number of clients
       that it should in line with the
       PRIP overall program aims and
       objectives?   _____

   1.2 <u>Potential for future</u>? What is
       the potential for the future
       growth of my unit (interest area)?   _____

   1.3 <u>Client loyalty</u>? How loyal are
       the present clients in my unit
       (interest area)?   _____

2. Competition:

   2.1 <u>Knowledge about competition #1</u>?
       How adequate is my knowledge about
       the <u>direct</u> competition that my unit
       (interest area) is facing? (i.e., other
       university-sponsored activities)   _____

   2.2 <u>Knowledge about competition #2</u>?
       How adequate is my knowledge about
       the <u>indirect</u> competition that my
       unit (interest area) is facing?
       (i.e., non-university-sponsored
       entertainment activities)   _____

   2.3 <u>Time scheduling</u>? If direct or
       indirect competition (i.e., other
       programs) are scheduled at the same
       time, how good are the chances that
       my unit (interest area) will be chosen?   _____

198

3. Knowledge of societal and/or environmental trends? How adequate is my knowledge and understanding of social, legal, political, and techno logical trends, etc. in relation to the present status of my unit (interest area)?   _____

4. Present market situation? Everything considered, how do I rate my unit's (interest area's) share of the presently available market?   _____

B. AVERAGE RATING--MARKET CAPABILITIES   = _____

C. ORGANIZATION'S (PRIP's) CAPABILITIES
   (from an overall standpoint)

1. Financial status?

   1.1 Ability to meet costs? Keeping the present situation in mind, how do I rate our ability to balance the budget each year?   _____

   1.2 University funding #1? How do I rate the adequacy of University funding based on what should be made available?   _____

   1.3 University funding #2? How do I rate the adequacy of University funding based on what is provided by universities for other PRIP programs within the OUAA?   _____

   1.4 Revenue generation #1? How do I assess the adequacy of the level to which program participants

contribute through basic activity/
membership fees to the support of PRIP? _____

1.5 <u>Revenue generation #2?</u> How do I
assess the adequacy of the level
to which program participants
contribute for special, expensive
program features and offerings? _____

2. How do I assess PRIP's (Program's)
adaptability (i.e. to expand
or to make revisions)? _____

3. How do I rate the overall PRIP
(Program) structure (i.e. its
balance and individual strengths)? _____

4. Personnel:

4.1 <u>Management personnel?</u> How
do I assess the management
of the overall program (i.e.,
generally and specifically)? _____

4.2 <u>Support Staff</u> How do I
evaluate the overall performance
of the various members of the
support staff? _____

4.3 <u>Part-Time Staff</u> How do I
evaluate the performance
of the part-time staff? _____

4.4 <u>Physical Plant Personnel</u> How do
I assess the maintenance services
provided by the staff in the
Physical Plant? _____

C. AVERAGE RATING--PRIP/PROGRAM STATUS   = _____

(Please add up the individual ratings you felt able to complete and then divide the total by the number of individual responses that you made [i.e., divide the total by the DIVISOR and enter the number obtained under C immediately above].)

STEP THREE: EVALUATION OF UNITS' MARKETING PLANS

Note: In Step Three base your evaluation on your involvement with a specific unit of the entire Program (PRIP).

Numerical
Score
(e.g., EX=5)

A. MARKET PENETRATION
(i.e., to what extent is my unit (interest area) under the PRIP working to increase the use of present services in the current markets?)

1. To increase the use of services by:

1.1 Advertising? Is the advertising for my unit (area of interest) sufficient quality and quantity _____

1.2 Price cutting? What is the adequacy of the price established for special services within my unit? _____

1.3 Promotional devices? How adequate are the promotional gimmicks or devices that are used in connection with my unit? _____

1.4 <u>Enhancing the benefits of parti-
cipation</u>? Are we currently offering service in such a way that the
benefits of participation in an
activity are being steadily enhanced?
(i.e., striving to "give more bang
for the buck")   _____

2. Attracting participants from other
units? Are our current efforts as
described in #1 immediately above
of such quality and quantity that
participants from other units (interest
areas) are joining my particular unit?   _____

3. Attracting current non-users? Are
our current efforts as described in #1
above of such quality and quantity
that current non-users of any PRIP
services are getting involved?   _____

B. MARKET DEVELOPMENT
(i.e., to what extent are the several
units (sub-programs under PRIP)
working to increase the use of
current services in <u>new</u> markets)

1. Capability to expand? (i.e., To what
extent does my unit (interest area)
have the <u>capability</u> to serve any
untapped new markets for the program
I represent?)

1.1 <u>University</u>? To what extent
does my unit (interest area)
have the capability to expand
on campus?   _____

1.2 <u>Alumni</u>? To what extent does my
unit (interest area) have the

capability to expand to serve
alumni within the 11 counties
that the UWO serves basically?

_____

1.2 <u>Local community</u>? To what extent
does my unit (interest area)
have the capability to expand to
the Greater London Area?

_____

2. Services that appeal to new segments
of potential markets? If services were
made available to new segments with
appropriate advertising, to what extent
might my unit (interest area) attract
new segments of the "populations"
mentioned immediately above?

_____

C. PRODUCT DEVELOPMENT & DIVERSIFICATION
(i.e., to what extent am I expanding [1]
present services for current markets and/or
[2] **new**, **dissimilar** services within my
unit (interest area) to attract new
classes of participants?)

<u>Present Product Development</u>

1. Have I the potential to adapt or modify
<u>present</u> services or activities within
within my unit (interest area)?
(e.g., fitness, intramurals)

_____

2. Have I the potential to create
<u>different levels</u> of services within
my unit (interest area)? (e.g., novice,
intermediate, and advanced levels)

_____

3. Have I the potential to develop <u>new</u>
services or activities for current
markets within my unit (interest
area)? (e.g., computerized stroke

analysis in golf instruction classes)? _____

New, Dissimilar Services

4. Describe the availability of facilities
   for new, dissimilar, types of activities
   within my unit (interest area) to attract
   new participants? (e.g., competitive water
   wrestling within aquatics) _____

5. Could I obtain supervisory personnel to
   develop new, dissimilar services? _____

6. Could I obtain instructors for new,
   dissimilar services? _____

D. INTEGRATIVE GROWTH
   (i.e., could I work to increase efficiency
   or unit (interest area) use by expanding or
   moving "backward, forward, or horizontally"
   within the target market [examples below]?)

1. Ability to control facility use? The
   extent to which I can control the use of
   facilities needed for my unit (interest
   area)? _____

2. Ability to control activities and
   scheduling for my unit (interest area)?
   The extent to which I have the freedom or
   leeway to make such program adjustments? _____

3. Ability to make input concerning other
   program units in the overall market area?
   The extent to which I can make input
   into the planning for other units
   within PRIP? _____

E. AVERAGE RATING OF GROWTH DIRECTIONS

OR FUNCTIONAL STRATEGIES WITHIN THE
OVERALL MARKETING PLAN DEVELOPMENT = _____

(Please add up the individual ratings you felt
able to complete and then divide the total by
the number of individual responses that you
made--i.e., divide the total by the DIVISOR
and enter the number obtained under E
immediately above.)

STEP FOUR: ASSESSMENT OF PRESENT UNIT MARKETING MIX

INSTRUCTIONS FOR DETERMINATION OF THE MARKETING MIX

The marketing mix can be regarded as the actual (recognized or
unrecognized) marketing plan presently in existence for the
overall program and its several sub-program components.

This Marketing Mix is the sum of the time, effort, and resources
expended on the present implementation of any functional
strategies currently employed.

It consists typically of four elements as follows: (1) PRODUCT, (2)
PLACE, (3) PROMOTION, and (4) PRICE.

An analysis of each of the four elements of the Unit Marketing Mix
(e.g., product, place) is a required step for future planning.

Once the weightings of the present aims, status, and functional
strategies have been determined, the results should be discussed
carefully.

Any relationship between the UNIT MARKETING MIX RATING
(STEP FOUR) and the rating(s) determined in STEPS ONE, TWO,
and THREE (including the OVERALL RATING AVERAGE) should
be discussed after the latter rating(s) have been established.

In all probability, there will be a close correlation between the MARKETING MIX RATING and the OVERALL RATING AVERAGE!

Decisions concerning any <u>future</u> Marketing Plan in keeping with the desired Marketing Mix may then be made at the end of the planning process.

Assessment of the established UNIT <u>and</u> PROGRAM Marketing Mix should be carried out periodically for best results (e.g., annually, biennially). Fine tuning may be required even sooner.

> <u>Note</u>: Here you are asked to assess the present marketing mix of your unit in the overall PRIP program.

<u>Numerical</u>
<u>Score</u>
(e.g., EXC=5)

A. PRODUCT

1. Overall quality of services offered? (ncluding instruction)   _____

2. Number of services or activities offered?   _____

3. Variety in the program offerings?   _____

4. General appeal to participants?   _____

5. Quality of <u>non-program</u> services offered?

   5.1 Locker rooms / reservations   _____

   5.2 Administrative / supervisory   _____
   5.3 Sports & Recreational Services

Office _____

B. PLACE

1. Locations of the services? _____

2. Access to services (e.g., overcrowding)? _____

3. Planning of services offered? _____

4. Quality of equipment? _____

5. Availability of facilities? _____

6. General atmosphere? _____

7. Homogeneity of attendees (where services dictate a need)? _____

C. PROMOTION

1. Public relations?

   1.1 With undergraduate students? _____

   1.2 With graduate students? _____

   1.3 With faculty members? _____

   1.4 With staff members? _____

   1.5 With alumni & larger community? _____

   1.6 With various media? _____

2. Personal selling of program? _____

3. Advertising (regular, paid)?

3.1 Variety of media used?   _____

3.2 Timing?   _____

3.3 Amount of advertising used?   _____

3.4 Quality of advertising
   "messages"?   _____

4. Advertising (<u>unpaid</u> exposure)?

                                               _____

5. Short-term promotions
   (e.g., special events)?   _____

D. PRICE

1. Amount of fees charged for
   <u>ongoing</u> services?   _____

2. Amount of fees charged for
   <u>special</u> services?   _____

3. Collection procedures?   _____

4. Discounts/allowances?   _____

5. Refunding policies?   _____

E. AVERAGE MARKETING MIX RATING   =   _____

   (Please add up the individual ratings you felt able
   to complete and then divide the total by the
   number of individual responses that you made--i.e.,
   divide the total by the DIVISOR and enter the
   number obtained under E immediately above.)

STEP FIVE: DETERMINATION OF A FUTURE MARKETING PLAN
(including a Revised Marketing Mix with Appropriate Financial Implications)

<u>Note</u>: At this point the entire group will become a Committee of the Whole to facilitate ready input and discussion.

The managers and the unit coordinators will be asked to form a panel of resource people at the front of the room. Others will be seated in a semi-circle facing the panel.

A marketing mix <u>outline</u> will be placed on a blackboard, and present finance and resource allocations in tabular or chart form will be made available to facilitate discussion.

The plan is to receive a variety of inputs from the various units and services (i.e., greatest strength and evident weakness) on the various headings under the Marketing Plan and the Marketing Mix as follows:

Marketing Plan	Marketing Mix
Market Penetration (increasing use of current features, services in <u>present</u> market) packaging,	**Product:** (quality, options, variety)
Market Development (increasing use of current timing, services in <u>new</u> markets) coverage)	**Place:** (locations, transport,
Product Development (developing <u>expanded</u> services	**Promotion** (advertising, selling,

for current markets)

media, special
events)

Diversification
(developing <u>new</u> dissimilar
refunds,
services for new markets)
payments)

Price/Fees
(allowances,

fee increases,

Integrative Growth
(increasing efficiency or
program use within current
market)

EVALUATION SCHEDULE SUMMARY

<u>Numerical</u>

<u>Score</u>

<u>STEP ONE</u>:   Definition of the Organization   _____
                    (OVERALL)

<u>STEP TWO</u>:   Status of the Organization   _____
                    (UNIT & OVERALL)

<u>STEP THREE</u>: Evaluation of the Present
                    Marketing Plan   _____
                    (UNIT)

<u>STEP FOUR</u>:   Assessment of the Present
                    Marketing Mix   _____
                    (UNIT)

<u>OVERALL AVERAGE RATING</u>
(FOR STEPS 1 THROUGH 4)   _____

<u>Note</u>: This final Overall Average Rating may be regarded in the same light as the individual ratings and average ratings of STEPS made throughout the evaluation process (from EX [5] down to PO [1]). (The entire process is still subjective, of course, but an evaluation adds rationality to this future planning exercise. Thank you for participating.

<u>STEP FIVE</u>: Determination of a Future Marketing Plan (including a Revised Marketing Mix with Appropriate Financial Implications)

<u>Recommendations</u> <u>from a Committee of the Whole</u>

<u>A Final Note</u>: You are not asked to sign your name to this evaluation. However, it would be helpful if you would indicate the unit within PRIP where you work. Please place an "<u>X</u>" alongside the appropriate unit. Thank you for your involvement in the day's evaluation sessions.

_____ Intramural Sports   _____ Casual Recreation

_____ Non-Credit Instruction   _____ Aquatics

_____ Fitness   _____ Sport Clubs

_____ General Administration   _____ Sports and Rec.
                                                   Services
                                                   (incl. locker room
                                                          staff)

Instructions:
Please help us evaluate the effectiveness of today's PRIP Retreat. Use the same numerical ratings that were followed on the Evaluation Schedule.

Evaluation

1. Did you develop some understanding of strategic market planning?...................... _____

2. Did you develop a better understanding of the entire PRIP program?..................... _____

3. Did you develop a better understanding of your own special area of involvement?........ _____

4. Did you have an opportunity to express your feelings and beliefs about the overall program and/or your own unit?........... _____

5. Do you think that PRIP's leadership will develop a better understanding about the program's future develop-ment after today's planning session?............ _____

6. Is leaving the campus for this planning session a good idea?............................ _____

7. How do you rate Spencer Lodge for this purpose?................................... _____

8. How do you rate the overall planning session?....................................... _____

9. What other thoughts do you have on this subject?

_____

_____

_____

PART 8
EVALUATION OF ADMINISTRATOR
BY FACULTY MEMBERS

Just about one hundred percent of those who may read these words have been involved with academic courses where teacher evaluation was carried out at the end of the course experience. Perhaps we can all agree that such evaluation is a good idea for several reasons. It would be interesting, however, to know how many teachers and professors have had the opportunity to evaluate the performance of their supervisors or department heads or chairpersons.

Throughout my career at the university level, when I was personally *not* the administrative head, I *never* had the opportunity to do so. As a believer in the institution of as much democracy as is humanly possible into academic units at the university level, I decided to do just that when I became a dean at The University of Western Ontario. The results were interesting and disappointing in some respects. Overall I suppose it can be stated that the execution of the plan was a "reasonable success." However, when I finally got to see the anonymous results for me as dean and for the several program administrators, it was disappointing to see that some people–despite the fact that great6 care was taken to preserve anonymity–didn't trust "the administration" to have carried the enterprise out anonymously. With selected other results, it turned out that some faculty members criticized why so-and-so as administrator had done such-and-such because they themselves "didn't know what was going on" (i.e., the particular faculty was ignorant of the fact that such-and-such a policy was in effect because the majority of faculty members had voted for it!

Overall, however, I think annual evaluation of the administrator or manager is a good idea–and I would carry such a policy out again if I were in a potion to do so.

(Please proceed to the next page)

APPRAISAL GUIDE FOR THE ADMINISTRATOR/MANAGER

developed by
Earle F. Zeigler, Ph.D.
The University of Western Ontario

Instructions (General)

It is quite common for faculty or staff members in educational institutions and other agencies to be evaluated in one or more ways by those who are selected to administer or manage. However, the converse--rating of administrative or managerial performance by faculty or staff--is not the case nearly as often. Why this continues to be so would make an interesting study in itself. Of course, it is quite possible that many public, semi-public, and private agencies are still not ready for the implementation of a plan of evaluation for managers (by workers) as well as for workers (by managers).

However, we do know that the organizational climate has been changing; thus, this appraisal guide is offered for consideration and possible use. Obviously, a concept of 'organizational democracy' should prevail for the institution of an appraisal such as this on a trial basis. Many administrators and managers, as well as many faculty and/or staff members, now agree that some mechanism should be devised to appraise the administrators/managers with whom they are primarily associated. (The investigator, when serving as an administrator in the mid-1970s, experimented with the idea of evaluation for all managerial personnel with good results.)

With any testing device or instrument, questions arises immediately as to the test's validity, reliability, and objectivity. Efforts are being made to answer these questions in the best way possible.

In considering the performance of the individual administrator or manager, the following characteristics, traits, execution of functions, etc. have been included:

1. Job Knowledge
2. Planning and Organizing Work
3. Supervisory Functions
4. Working with People
5. Personal Traits
6. Drive and Initiative
7. Cooperation and Team play

As you begin this evaluation, please keep in mind that the administrator is typically required (expected?) to have the following types of <u>knowledge</u>, <u>competencies</u>, and <u>skills</u>: personal, conceptual, human, and technical (Katz). Also, the administrative <u>process</u> is typically viewed as involving planning, organizing, staffing, directing, and controlling (i.e., ensuring that all is progressing normally according to plan) (Mackenzie).

In assessing any administrator/manager, the evaluation should be based primarily on whether he or she has fulfilled the responsibilities and duties of the post capably. *Those who are appraising the managerial efforts of another should be aware of the agreed-upon job description for the position.* In many cases this has been spelled out carefully and is available for all to examine. Thus, you are assessing administrative performance not so much on the basis of <u>your own personal idea</u> of how the job should be done, but more on what it is generally expected (i.e., the job description and existing institutional rules and regulations) that the manager executes to fulfill his or her duties and responsibilities.

Instructions (Specific)

In this Appraisal Guide for the Administrator/Manager, therefore, you will find twenty (20) questions covering different phases of a person's job performance. These questions were gleaned from various sources in the literature, with the questionnaire format itself adapted initially from a format developed by General Telephone System (n.d.).

Please place an "X" in the appropriate box before the adjective (Excellent, Good, Fair, Poor, X) that most nearly answers the question asked. You should do this by judging how adequately the administrator measures up to his or her present job responsibilities and duties. Thus, you should considered carefully what the job is, its degree of responsibility, its degree of authority, how it fits into the organization, and what kind of person is required. <u>If you don't know</u>, ask questions to get answers to aspects of the post you don't know or understand. If you really do not have enough information to answer a question accurately (and you can't locate the answer), indicate that you "cannot form a judgment based on experience" (X).

Understand that your response to this questionnaire will remain absolutely anonymous (no identifying numbers are included anywhere). *This puts unusual pressure upon you to be fair and ethical to the best of your ability (and conscience!).* The plan in using this appraisal form is to make two ratings available to all members of the faculty and staff: (1) the numerical average from the <u>one</u> General Overall Rating requested at the end of the questionnaire (e.g., 3.3), and (2) the overall numerical average of the 20 individual items added together and averaged (e.g., 3.4). This should suffice

to let faculty and/or staff members know how the final, subjective, overall assessment each person offered
compares to the average evaluation of his or her peers determined in two ways (as explained above).

The administrator, however, would receive the results of the 20 item-by-item evaluations along with two overall assessments, the one determined from the overall subjective assessment and the other the overall averaging of the 20 individual-item averages. The manager would also receive a summary of any other comments offered in the open-ended section of each individual questionnaire.

Please place the completed questionnaire unsigned and sealed in the blank white envelope in the sealed carton provided in the administrator's office during regular office hours. The secretary on duty will check your name off on a roster indicating that you have "voted." This must be done before [say] June 15 at 1:30 p.m.

A tally and summary of the returns will be prepared subsequently by a committee of three determined by faculty/staff ballot, which in turn shall name its own chairperson at its first meeting prior to fulfilling its function. The results will remain confidential as to <u>specifics</u>, but the Executive Committee will be notified officially by the committee chairperson as to the two numerical averages as explained above. The Executive Committee will not see the synopsis of the final individual comments, nor any other results of the averages of specific categories within the appraisal guide. Within a month the committee chairperson shall shred all returns in the presence of the administrator concerned.

Note: Please consider it your professional responsibility to complete this evaluation and turn it in prior to the deadline established. To be fair to the administrator/manager, it is important that we obtain as close as possible to a 100% return. Thank you.

Keep in mind that an <u>Excellent</u> evaluation means an assessment ranging from 3.1 to 4.0, a <u>Good</u> ranges from 2.1 to 3.0, a <u>Fair</u> ranges from 1.1 to 2.0, and a <u>Poor</u> ranges from 0 to 1.0.

Name of Person Being Evaluated _____

I. Can the administrator get ideas across to other people?

( ) Excellent = Expresses self well in speech and writing
( ) Good = Generally good; has some minor problems

216

( ) Fair = Has difficulties in communicating ideas
( ) Poor = Lacks skill in communication; often misunderstood
( ) X = Cannot form a judgment based on experience

II. Can the manager determine priorities with the tasks to be performed?

( ) Excellent = Yes; puts first things first
( ) Good = Usually takes care of the most important items
( ) Fair = To a degree; quite often concentrates on secondary items
( ) Poor = No; frequently spends time on items of little importance
( ) X = Cannot form a judgment based on experience

I
II. What is administrator's knowledge of present responsibility?

( ) Excellent = Full working knowledge of all major items
( ) Good = Good overall knowledge with a few weak spots
( ) Fair = Satisfactory knowledge with some definite gaps
( ) Poor = Does not have adequate job knowledge
( ) X = Cannot form an judgment based on experience

IV. Is manager a creative thinker?

( ) Excellent = Yes; uses original thought to solve problems often
( ) Good = Yes; can generally modify old ideas to meet new problems
( ) Fair = Not usually; shows very little creative thought
( ) Poor = No; usually follows former pattern or regulation
( ) X = Cannot form a judgment based on experience

V. Does manager consistently seek to build strong associates?

( ) Excellent = Yes; encourages variety of experiences for
        associates and gives ample opportunity to "get your
        feet wet"
( ) Good = Yes; most of the time staff members have varied assign-
    ments within the scope of their positions'
    responsibilities
( ) Fair = Somewhat; people are occasionally encouraged to accept
    new responsibilities or to volunteer for assignments
( ) Poor = No; assignments are far too rigid and tend to be
    stifling because the administrator dominates and holds
    people back
( ) X = Cannot form a judgment based on experience

VI. Can administrator accept criticism?

( ) Excellent = Takes fair criticism well; tries hard to improve
         thereafter
( ) Good = Accepts criticism favorably most of the time
( ) Fair = Not too well; is quite apt to resent it
( ) Poor = No; ignores it and often becomes quite disturbed
( ) X = Cannot form a judgment based on experience

VII. Is manager loyal to organizational policy once established?

( ) Excellent = Completely so, even when he/she disagrees
( ) Good = Will defend the organization's policy on most items
( ) Fair = Will often blame organization's policy for an unpopular
         procedure that manager must enforce
( ) Poor = Will enforce established policy only if he/she agrees
         with it
( ) X. Cannot form a judgment based on experience

VIII. .Has manager gained acceptance and "worn well" with staff?

( ) Excellent = Yes, the longer he/she is on the job, the greater
         the acceptance by the staff
( ) Good = Yes, he/she gets along very well most of the time
( ) Fair = Quite average; does have problems on a continuing basis
( ) Poor = Below average; has caused continuing irritation to a
         fair number of people
( )X. Cannot form a judgment based on experience

IX. Is the administrator a self-starter with initiative?

( ) Excellent = Yes; needs no urging to "get going" by
         himself/herself
( ) Good = Generally good; occasionally needs prodding or
         encouragement
( ) Fair = Often slow to get moving on own initiative
( ) Poor = Will react usually only if pressure is brought to bear
( ) X = Cannot form a judgment based on experience

X. Does manager systematically plan and complete work on schedule?

( ) Excellent = Consistently well organized and on schedule
( ) Good = Yes, typically plans well and generally on schedule
( ) Fair = Impression is created that forward planning is average;
         there is often rushing to meet deadlines
( ) Poor = A poor planner typically; often far behind in work
         schedule

( ) X = Cannot form a judgment based on experience

XI. How well does manager combine theoretical and practical ideas?

( ) Excellent = Combines both very effectively
( ) Good = Quite well, with occasional overemphasis one way
      or the other
( ) Fair = Average; there is some inability to preserve a balance
      on occasion
( ) Poor = Often significant overemphasis in one direction or the
      other
( ) X = Cannot form a judgment based on experience

XII. Does manager control his/her anger?

( ) Excellent = Maintains firm self-control
( ) Good = Almost always; on occasion gets excited
( ) Fair = Fairly well; needs to exercise more self-control
( ) Poor = Apt to blow up at any given moment
( ) X = Cannot form a judgment based on experience

XIII. Does administrator make a good initial impression?

( ) Excellent = Yes; people like him/her at once
( ) Good = People take to him quite soon
( ) Fair = So-so; sometimes creates an unfavorable impression
( ) Poor = Generally makes a poor first impression
( ) X = Cannot form a judgment based on experience

XIV. How well does manager understand the organization's general
     policies and procedures?

( ) Excellent = Full working knowledge of most major items
( ) Good = Quite good overall knowledge; has some weak spots
( ) Fair = Present knowledge is just enough to get the job done
( ) Poor = Needs considerable amount of study and/or training to
      develop adequate knowledge
( ) X = Cannot form a judgment based on experience

XV. Is manager open-minded in considering new ideas?

( ) Excellent = Freely accepts new ideas for consideration
( ) Good = Quite open-minded; occasionally seeks to avoid an idea
      because of source
( ) Fair = Somewhat open-minded, but has some problems here
( ) Poor = Considers new ideas if they are his own (or he "co-opts"
      them from someone else); otherwise forget it!

( ) X = Cannot form a judgment based on experience

XVI. Is administrator honest and above board in dealing with people?

  ( ) Excellent = Completely honest, dependable, and reliable
  ( ) Good = Typically honest and dependable
  ( ) Fair = Fairly good; occasionally has problems here
  ( ) Poor = Quite unreliable; often gives concern
  ( ) X = Cannot form a judgment based on experience

XVII. Does manager follow the organizational channels?

  ( ) Excellent = Carefully follows proper channels in his/her work
  ( ) Good = Usually goes through proper channels
  ( ) Fair = Quite often; occasionally takes "short cuts"
  ( ) Poor = Tends to create tensions quite often because he/she does
          not follow organizational channels
  ( ) X = Cannot form a judgment based on experience

XVIII. How fast and sound a thinker is he/she?

  ( ) Excellent = Has a "rapid" mind that quickly develops sound
            thoughts and progressions
  ( ) Good = Quite fast; typically does well in this regard
  ( ) Fair = Pretty good; occasionally makes leaps to conclusions
  ( ) Poor = You can hear the wheels grinding, and the response is
          usually not on the beam
  ( ) X = Cannot form a judgment based on experience

XIX. How capable is the manager in imparting knowledge to others?

  ( ) Excellent = An excellent teacher; imparts knowledge effectively
  ( ) Good = A good teacher; generally most satisfactory
  ( ) Fair = Fairly good, but has some weaknesses
  ( ) Poor = Does a poor teaching job
  ( ) X = Cannot form a judgment based on experience

XX. Is administrator willing to work along with the decision-making
     process operative within the organization?

  ( ) Excellent = Yes, in all regards
  ( ) Good = Generally he/she is, with occasional lapses
  ( ) Fair = Quite well, but the process is often painful to him/her
  ( ) Poor = Not really; participatory democracy would give him/her
          an ulcer
  ( ) X = Cannot form a judgment based on experience

General Overall Rating

Everything considered. this person should receive the following rating for the administrative/managerial work he/she is currently carrying out within the organization:

( ) Excellent

( ) Good

( ) Fair

( ) Poor

Thank you for completing this questionnaire. If there is anything else you would like to say, please write it immediately below.

_____

_____

_____

_____

_____

_____

PART 9
EVALUATING LIFE'S LEISURE COMPONENT

The field known as physical (activity) education, kinesiology, sport management (or whatever...) has chosen in various circumstances to call itself a profession, a discipline, a quasi-discipline. It can be also be argued that physical education is a subject within professional education when it is subsumed under that category. Whatever the case may be, or however you decide what you think should be the case, we have many adherents who take themselves too seriously and may well be called fanatics because of their almost incessant involvement with teaching and coaching.

With this thought in mind some years ago, I decided to devise a way whereby men and women professionals might carry out a self-evaluation of their "RQ" or recreation quotient. In 2002 I expanded this undertaking into a book titled *Whatever happened to "The Good Life"? (Assessing your "RQ" (recreation quotient)*. Subsequently it was published in India, as well as Bloomington, Indiana.

You are urged to test yourself in this regard. Although the findings about yourself can be meaningful, the testing should be carried out in a light-hearted manner. Nevertheless, you may find that the results offer "solid food for digestion." Each of us gets only "one shot" at leading "The Good Life". We should choose how we spend our time wisely.

Please move a head to Page 223

A TEST FOR SELF-EVALUATION
OF YOUR "RQ" (RECREATION QUOTIENT)

Earle F. Zeigler, Ph.D.

Throughout history many societies misused leisure after they have earned it. In some instances the misuse of free time actually caused the downfall of that society.

North Americans have been accused of having spectatoritis—that is, spending too much of their free time watching others taking part in some form of recreation.

Many people are concerned about whether they are getting sufficient pleasure out of life. Here is an opportunity to determine your overall "recreational quotient" based on involvement (or lack of same) in a variety of recreational pursuits.

This simple, self-evaluative test for adults of all ages was developed so that men and women could rate themselves recreationally and then take steps as they wish to improve their "recreational quotient." There is no doubt but that sound recreational pursuits can add zest and vigor to our lives.

We can appreciate that there are many ways of looking at the area of recreation. However, although we could determine averages (or norms) for a given population as to types of recreational pursuits followed, it doesn't seem advisable to set standards in a free society.

Of course, one development of modern society has been that people are increasingly crowded together in heavily populated urban and suburban communities. This creates a problem: How can people find happiness, satisfaction, and a high quality of life despite and increased tempo of living and increasing crowded conditions?

In taking this test—i.e., carrying out this self-evaluation—please answer the questions as honestly and frankly as possible. The test is based on a scale moving from passive, to vicarious, to active, to creative involvement in life's educational and recreational activities. It gives you more credit if you are a most interested onlooker or listener rather than a passive one. Moreover, you will score even higher if you actively take part in a particular recreational activity. The highest rating goes to the person who participates in a superior and/or creative fashion. Instructions

Give yourself one point if you answer "yes" to question no.1 under sport and physical recreational interests. In like manner give yourself two points for answering question no. 2 affirmatively, three points for question no. 3, and four points for no. 4. The maximum score for each category is ten points.

At the bottom of each section (or category of recreational interest), total your score from each of the four questions in that section. When you have completed all of the questions in the five categories, total the scores from the different categories.

Finally, rate yourself according to the scale for your grand total, and also according to the scale for individual sections. Although in developing this self-evaluation scale, we did give you more points for active involvement, we are not seeking to establish an overall standard for participation.

After you have completed this assessment and determined your recreation quotient ("RQ"), we will offer some suggestions and recommendations for your consideration. (Please begin now on the next page.)

CATEGORY 1

Sports and Physical Activity
(e.g., golf, bowling, exercise class, walking)

1.   Do you regularly at least glance through the sports section of your local newspaper?

Yes ( ) or No ( )..................... Score _____

2. Are you a faithful follower of at least one team or athlete, rejoicing in victory and fretting in defeat?

Yes ( ) or No ( )..................... Score _____

3. Do you take part at least two or three times a week through-out the entire in regular physical activity (e.g., an active game or sport, brisk walking for a mile)

Yes ( ) or No ( )..................... Score _____

4. Are you considered one of the better players in any active physical activity or active game or sport among opponents your own age?

Yes ( ) or No ( )..................... Score _____

Total Score for this Section................ Score _____

Scale: 10 pts. —- superior; 6 pts. —- good; 3 pts. —- fair; 1 pt. —- poor

CATEGORY 2

Social Activities
(e.g., social club, church
outing, family recreation)

1. Do you take pleasure in make nodding acquaintances and exchanging
    the time of day with a number of people?

Yes ( ) or No ( )..................... Score _____

2. Do you take an interest in and attend at least one social club or organization regularly?

Yes ( ) or No ( )..................... Score _____

3. Do you invite friends in for dinner or a social get-together

(or invite someone out) at least once a month?

Yes ( ) or No ( )..................... Score _____

4. In the past year have you been elected an officer or served
   as a committee chairperson of a club or a social or political
   organization?

Yes ( ) or No ( )..................... Score _____

Total Score for this Section................ Score _____

Scale: 10 pts. — superior; 6 pts. — good; 3 pts. — fair; 1 pt. — poor

CATEGORY 3

Communicative Activities
(e.g., article writing, letter
to editor, speaking, discussions)

1. Do you telephone or drop in on a friend regularly just to pass
   the time of day?

Yes ( ) or No ( )..................... Score _____

2. Do you argue for a point of view even though it may mean a
   difference of opinion with a close friend or committee
   chairperson?

Yes ( ) or No ( )..................... Score _____

3. Have you in the past six months written one or more letters
   strongly expressing your opinion to an editor, school
principal,
   or civic official?

Yes ( ) or No ( )..................... Score _____

4. In the past year have you given a talk or led discussion at
   your PTA, church, or any other local group?

Yes ( ) or No ( )..................... Score _____

Total Score for this Section................ Score _____

(See scale under Categories 1 & 2 above)

CATEGORY 4

Aesthetic & Creative Activities ("Cultural")
(e.g., oil painting, music, sculpting)

1. Do you like to listen to a musical concert or watch a serious drama on television?

Yes ( ) or No ( )..................... Score _____

2. Have you attended at least three or four concerts, play, or art exhibits in the past year?

Yes ( ) or No ( )..................... Score _____

3. Do you paint, sketch, play an instrument, or sing, etc. regularly?

Yes ( ) or No ( )..................... Score _____

4. If your answer to #3 immediately above, do you rate yourself sufficiently high to enter a content or competition?

Yes ( ) or No ( )..................... Score _____

Total Score for this Section................ Score _____

(See scale under Categories 1 & 2 above)

CATEGORY 5

Educational Activities
(e.g., hobbies: ham radio, gardening,

astronomy, coin-collecting)

1. Do you like to hear or read about the learning interests of
   others?

Yes ( ) or No ( )..................... Score _____

2. Are you so interested and knowledgeable in any educational or
   recreational hobby (apart from one you are engaged in
yourself)
   that you could discuss it intelligently with an expert on the
subject?

Yes ( ) or No ( )..................... Score _____

3. Do you have a "learning-interest" hobby of your own in which
   you are involved regularly?

Yes ( ) or No ( )..................... Score _____

4. Are you considered an expert on your hobby, one to whom
others
   may turn for advice, and possibly having won an award or
special
   mention in the past year or two?

Yes ( ) or No ( )..................... Score _____

Total Score for this Section............... Score _____

(See scale under Categories 1 & 2 above)

NOW ADD UP THE TOTAL FOR EACH CATEGORY TO GET
YOUR
GRAND TOTAL.

                                    YOUR FINAL SCORE =

_____

ANALYSIS:

Now rate yourself according to the following scale:

50-35 pts.—Outstanding—You may be getting too much fun and pleasure out of life. How about doing some more constructive work for a change?

34-24 pts.—Above Average—You may have achieved a balance between work and play in your life. You are evidently enjoying your leisure without having a guilty conscience.

23-14 pts.—Average—Your score indicate a fair status. You may be somewhat narrow or one-sided, or you may not have achieved much depth in anything. Check this out keeping the ideal in mind.

13-6 pts.—Below Average—You are missing some of the good things, the pleasurable activities, that life has to offer. Review and assess your goals for living.

5-0 pts.—Poor—Life is undoubtedly a tedious routine for you. Wake up and live!

RECOMMENDATIONS / SUGGESTIONS

This assessment of your personal "recreational quotient," obviously a subjective evaluation (plus an attempt to be a bit humorous), is based on the premise that you should determine intelligently and carefully what it is that you want out of life. What do you value in your life?

Some might say they want pleasure, knowledge, and prestige, while others might stress creativity, adventure, and good health. A third group might wish for improvement of certain personality traits, a renewal of religious faith, and a continued capacity to profit from a lifelong education.

However you may rank your personal values in descending order, there is solid evidence that choosing a sound educational/recreational pattern in your life is difficult and should be an ever-changing challenge throughout life. The premise upon which this test is based is that the specific decisions you make about which free-time activities you will be involved with—and how you go about carrying them out—can mean a great deal toward the achievement of your life goals.

Some people are lucky enough to have a career in which they can find the satisfactions which coincide with many of their chosen values. But you may not a position where this is possible. This is why it is so important for you to establish your own hierarchy of values and then to select your educational/recreational pattern of living. We wish you well in this quest. . . .

Part 10
Balancing Life's Conflicting Aspects:
A Challenge for the Sport
and Physical Activity Administrator

(Author's Note: This background essay is intended to be synoptic in nature. It represents an evolving version of many of the ideas, opinions, and recommendations expressed by the author about management theory and practice as applied to physical education and sport in a variety of publications over a period of approximately 60years. Prior to a collaborative effort with Gary Bowie (University of Lethbridge) designed to introduce a management competency development approach to professional preparation in physical education and educational sport, the author had collaborated earlier, also, with Marcia Spaeth (retired from SUNY, Cortland) and Garth Paton and Terry Haggerty (now both at New Brunswick, but earlier at Western Ontario). Some of this material (i.e., that related to proposed areas of administrative research and that related to the professional preparation program) had been researched by Professor Spaeth and Professor Paton, respectively and appeared in Zeigler and Spaeth [1975]).

Introduction

In this chapter I hope to bring this dilemma down to the personal level. It is an effort to get you, the reader, to figure out-- unless you are absolutely certain where you stand on the matter already–where you may be going in the years ahead in a field that is uncertain as well. Nevertheless, translating the disciplinary theory of "kinesiology" into generalizations about professional practice in physical activity education is fundamentally important to our society. The lives of people of all ages and conditions can be affected positively if this aim is carried out efficiently and effectively. Our task in the field today is to discover a host of young Canadians who will "make things happen" so that the field of developmental physical activity will prosper and thereby fulfill the potential for humankind that it inherently offers.

The purpose of this analysis was to outline how a sport and physical activity administrator (e.g., of physical activity education & athletics) might better comprehend the need to balance life's "conflicting aspects." These conflicting aspects are typically the broadening of one's professional vision while simultaneously seeking to maintain perspective as to his or her chosen aims and objectives in life. It was decided to employ a systems analysis approach to help explain what can be called "human and natural (or physical) ecologic interaction." The main problem of the analysis was first divided into five sub-problems (phrased as questions) for subsequent consideration:

1. Why should an administrator of physical activity education (including athletics) understand the various ramifications of ecology for humankind?
2. How can systems analysis coordinated with "human and natural ecologic interaction" apply to the *organizational* task? of such an administrator?
3. How can systems analysis coordinated with human and natural ecological interaction apply to the *personal* development of this administrator?
4. How can the two approaches be merged to achieve both *successful professional* life and a *fulfilling personal* life?
5. What may be reasonably concluded from this discussion?

A Physical Activity Administrator Should Understand the Ramifications of Ecology for Humankind?

For this analysis, ecology was defined as "the field of study that treats the relationships and interactions of human beings and other living organisms with each other and with their natural (or physical) environment" (Hawley, 1986, p. 2). Ecology, which is much more than so-called "environmentalism," is about truly understanding relationships with and/or interactions between humans and other organisms within the environment. This involvement has no doubt been with humankind over the centuries. In addition, the apparent continuing lack of understanding and full appreciation of it by leaders, not to mention almost all others, has still not been overcome. Further, the steadily increasing size of the world's population and the accompanying vast societal development has exacerbated the problem even further.

To put the matter more simply, the basic underlying issue of dwindling supply and increasing demand has never been brought home sufficiently to the world's leadership, much less to the majority of the people. And, in the relatively few cases where it has, urgent *present* need has almost invariably thrust the need for preparation to meet impending *future* disasters aside. In fact, that appears to be exactly what is happening at this very time.

Despite the ever-increasing importance of this subject to humankind, somehow the vital importance of the subject of ecology as a *fundamental social institution* such as economics, politics, etc. did not begin to receive serious attention by at least a segment of society until the early 1960s.

Today, however, selected countries and certain groups within these countries are striving to come to grips with the need to face up to the headlong collision looming between ecology and economics as conflicting social forces. For example, Epstein (1997) reported that "five years after 10,000 diplomats from 178 countries pledged to clean up the world at the United Nations-sponsored Rio Earth Summit, the first formal assessment of that pledge begins today" (March 13). At the same session, Maurice Strong, the 1992 conference chair, stated: "the process of deterioration has continued..."

Since 1970, many educators have gradually come to understand that the problem of ecology was here to stay. Zeigler (1989; 2003), for example, designated it as a persistent problem faced by the field of sport and physical education in the same way as he had identified the five other basic social forces (or influences) of values, politics, nationalism, economics, and religion back in 1964. No longer, as it had almost always been possible in the past, could people simply move elsewhere to locate another abundant supply of game to hunt, water to drink, or mineral resources to exploit when on-site resources are depleted.

Today, as this problem is gradually being recognized globally with seemingly little response, the time is past due for the profession of physical education and sport to also pay special attention to this social force in the various aspects of its work.

More specifically, there are several very important reasons right now for the field to show ever-greater awareness of *human ecologic interaction* with its many ramifications for humankind. First, the promotion and subsequent development of such an awareness could soon result in the field's general acceptance of an overall human and natural (physical) ecologic orientation that could be designed to underlie all of its professional efforts. Such awareness and subsequent orientation would call the profession's attention to the fact that our basic concern as part-time and full-time administrators should be with the *total* life cycle of people considered both individually and collectively.

Second, the graduates of professional education programs, who subsequently serve as administrators or managers in organizations of all types functioning in culturally influenced environments, need to be so prepared they will understand and then commit themselves to the application of an overall ecological approach in their work. In this context this means that they, as professional managers serving as administrators, have a basic responsibility to develop and strengthen their particular institution or organization in which they serve so that it will have an ongoing capability *to adapt successfully to the changing (natural and cultural) environment in which it is located.*

They need to keep in mind that fundamental changes in society are continually taking place, and that they are accordingly influencing professionals in their administrative endeavor positively, negatively, or possibly not at all. This means that, at the practitioner's level, they should be (must be?) ever ready to meet such change (or lack of it) directly and adapt to it successfully if and when it occurs. For example, there appears to be an ever-present need to understand "cutback management" (or "management in decline," as it is often called. This, and other approaches are often called on in today's rapidly shifting environment. Another very important understanding that can

234

serve all administrators well is a reasonably basic comprehension of change process itself, a development that is ever present and requires the ongoing attention of the administrator.

Coordinating Systems Analysis with Human and Natural Ecologic Interaction in the the *Organizational* Task of the Administrator??

The scope of the systems function in management today has gone far beyond the dreams of the "scientific management" pioneers such as Taylor, the Gilbreths, and Henri Fayol. Today the sport management profession should be fully aware of the potentialities of an ongoing systems analysis approach. Such an approach should be *coordinated with* the best type of overall human and natural (physical) ecologic interaction as the profession seeks to serve the public professionally through the medium of sport and physical activity. Concurrently, in this analysis of the *professional* function (i.e., organizational "task") of the manager, the same systems-approach concept can be merged with overall human ecologic interaction as applied to the sport manager's *personal* development.

The first consideration here is with the intricacies of a systems approach that give attention to *how* this can be done most efficiently. The assumption behind a systems approach to human and natural ecologic interaction is that the physical activity-delivery organization and its administrator(s)--and the people functioning within it as associates--should all understand the importance and ramifications of a complete ecological approach and be committed to its implementation in all aspects of their work. If this were understood fully, they would then strive to serve their clients and constituents in ways that help the organization grow and develop. (At this point there will not be an explanation of *why* the administrator should strive for *general* aims in an ever-changing human and natural environment, or *what* specific objectives might be subsumed under these long range aims.)

With such an approach to management, the managerial team and key associated personnel would seek to develop, employ, and maintain power and influence that lead to the achievement of planned (immediate) objectives en route to long-range aims or goals. In doing so, they should involve many people within the organization in one way or another in assisting with the implementation of the well-recognized, fundamental processes of planning, organizing, staffing, directing, and controlling the operation of the organization (Mackenzie, 1969, pp. 80-87). Throughout this series of experiences it is imperative that good human relations be employed by all through the use of effective and efficient communication techniques. The successful implementation of these various processes is extremely complex, of course. This is why a top-flight managerial team is becoming increasingly necessary to move a complex organization ahead.

The major responsibilities of physical activity administrators (in physical education and sport), presuming they live up a code of ethics, should include:

(1) the professional's obligations to provide services to all in society who want and need them;

(2) the professional's specific obligations to his/her students/clients as individuals;

(3) the professional's responsibilities to his/her employers/employing organization;

(4) the professional's obligations to his colleagues/peers and to the profession; and

(5) the professional's responsibility to overall society itself (as recommended by Bayles in (Zeigler, 1992, pp. 13-14).

Figure 1
A Systems Model Describing Human Ecologic Interaction
for the Manager of Sport and Physical Activity

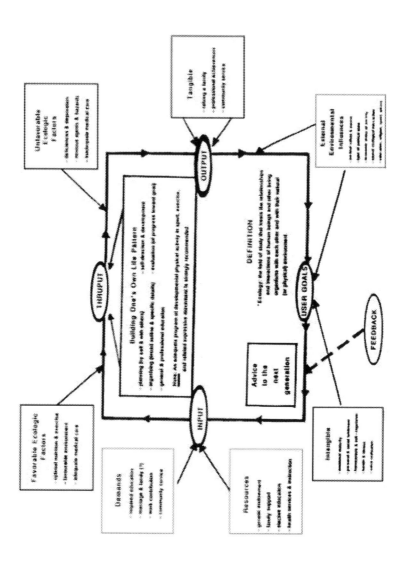

All of these obligations should be deliberately included in a code of ethics along with a procedure for disciplinary action to guarantee the enforcement of these responsibilities. (The latter procedure rarely been enforced in any profession to date--with notable exceptions [e.g., medicine, law, psychology]. Several professions have at least made some effort to discipline those colleagues who are reported as having acted unprofessionally and unethically. If a professional acts *illegally* within a given legal jurisdiction, it can, of course, be expected that the political jurisdiction itself will judge the severity of such action and make an appropriate decision. Such a decision will subsequently give guidance to a professional society's committee on ethics as to any disciplinary action it should take.)

To meet these professional obligations, the physical activity administrator will be involved both professionally and personally in an ongoing struggle for recognition and accompanying status as he/she fulfills (1) those important obligations that relate to his/her *professional* life, as well as (2) those obligations that are required for optimum *personal* development. Moving on, it will now be considered first how a schematic, systems-analysis model could assist the manager to comprehend fully the scope and intent of these obligations and/or responsibilities in both "realms" of his or her existence.

A Schematic Model for the Administrative Process That Embodies a Systems Approach

A generation ago a schematic model for the management process was developed (the elements of the set, so to speak) that arranged the elements of a systems approach logically within a behavioral science perspective (Milstein and Belasco, 1973). The concern was with *input, thruput,* and *output*, and it was stressed that these three aspects must be strongly interrelated because any systems outputs "that result from transforming the human and material resources within the educational system must be at least minimally acceptable to environmental groups and organizations" (p. 81). If the outputs are not acceptable, the external groups and organizations will quite simply let it be known in short order that the "lifeline" of human and material resources will be sharply cut or eliminated.

A schematic model of such a systems model is offered here, in this case a systems model for managerial effectiveness with a professional training program for physical activity administrators. Here the goal or output for the purpose of this discussion is related to the education of people for various careers relating to our field. It is a substantive adaptation of the material available in both Milstein and Belasco (1973) and George (1972). (See Figure 1 above.)

One definition of administration states that it involves the execution of managerial acts by a competent person, including the application of personal, interpersonal, conceptual, technical, and conjoined skills, while combining varying degrees of planning, organizing, staffing, directing (i.e., leading), and controlling (i.e., evaluation) within the management process to assist an organization to achieve its goals effectively and efficiently (Zeigler and Bowie, 1995, p. 115).

Further, the assumption is that such managerial acts will be directed toward individual and group goals within both the internal and external environments of an organization. In this example (Fig. 1), those directing the professional preparation program within a college or university perceive certain societal demands and/or needs (e.g., a societal demand for various types of physical activity administrators). Depending on the specific circumstance, the university and its alumni and supporters respond by making available (initially or potentially) (1) material and human resources such as available capital, (2) some level of achievement in sport competition and fitness promotion, and (3) a management program staff of good, bad, or indifferent stature. All of this initial development is, of course, ultimately part of the total administrative process itself. After the initial input stage has been started, we are really describing functions that occur within the larger management process that is typically characterized by such terms as planning, organizing, staffing, directing, and controlling (Mackenzie, 1969). For the administrator to execute these functions adequately, he or she should have acquired the

Figure 2

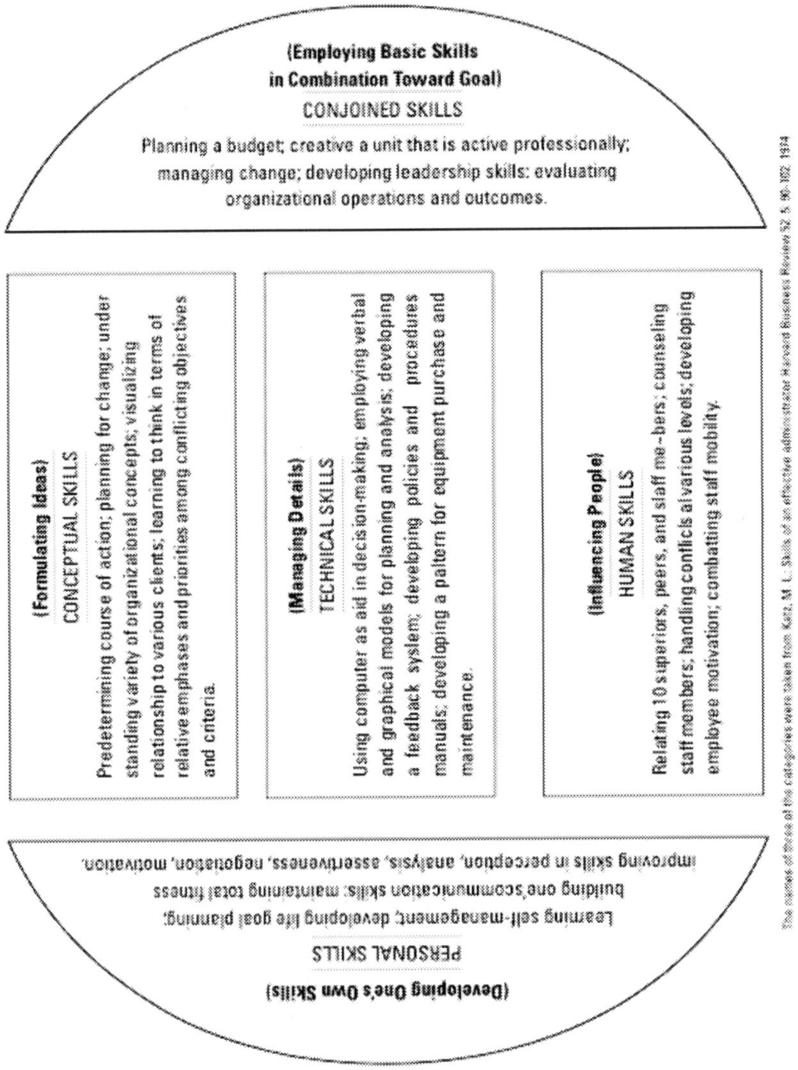

**(Employing Basic Skills
in Combination Toward Goal)**

CONJOINED SKILLS

Planning a budget; creative a unit that is active professionally;
managing change; developing leadership skills; evaluating
organizational operations and outcomes.

(Formulating Ideas)

CONCEPTUAL SKILLS

Predetermining course of action; planning for change; under
standing variety of organizational concepts; visualizing
relationship to various clients; learning to think in terms of
relative emphases and priorities among conflicting objectives
and criteria.

(Managing Details)

TECHNICAL SKILLS

Using computer as aid in decision-making; employing verbal
and graphical models for planning and analysis; developing
a feedback system; developing policies and procedures
manuals; developing a pattern for equipment purchase and
maintenance.

(Influencing People)

HUMAN SKILLS

Relating to superiors, peers, and staff me¬bers; counseling
staff members; handling conflicts at various levels; developing
employee motivation; combating staff mobility.

(Developing One's Own Skills)

PERSONAL SKILLS

Learning self-management; developing life goal planning;
building one'scommunication skills; maintaining total fitness
improving skills in perception, analysis, assertiveness, negotiation, motivation.

The sources of those of this categories were taken from Katz, M. L. Skills of an effective administrator Harvard Business Review 52 & 90-102, 1974

Management Development and Process (The knowledge and skills obtained through a competency-based approach).

necessary knowledge, competencies and skills (adapted from Katz, 1974, with advice from William Penny).

Thinking of the total administrative or managerial process in this example of a system analysis model for maximum effectiveness, keep in mind that there can be three categories of parameters and/or variables that influence the entire undertaking, as follows: (1) environmental *non controllable* parameters (constraints *or* opportunities), (2) internal *controllable* variables, and (3) *partially controllable* variables (that may be external and/or internal). It is important that physical activity administrators understand how strong these variables (influences) may be and accordingly be ever ready to factor their impact into the overall administrative process. Too often it appears that when such a non controllable or partially controllable parameter looms suddenly on the horizon, "internal panic" results because administrators-- and thus their organizations, of course--have not planned ahead and typically are *in no way* ready for its appearance.

The environmental *non–controllable* parameters should be viewed as external influences that must be considered seriously. They are such persistent historical problems as (1) the influence of the society's values and norms; (2) the influence of politics (the type of political state and the "stance" of the party or person in power); (3) the influence of nationalism (or whatever powerful "chauvinistic" influence might develop); (4) the influence of the prevailing economic situation (including depressions, tax increases, inflation, etc.); (5) the influence of prevailing religious groups (including boycotts, conflicting events); (6) the influence of ecology (as discussed above in this paper); and (7) the influence of competition (from other attractions, etc.).

To understand the concept of "administrative effectiveness" generally, as diagrammed in the model (Figure 1), it is necessary to consider specifically the relationship of managerial acts (ACTS) and the external and internal environments (Ee and Ei, respectively) of the organization to the eventual accomplishment of *at least a certain percentage* of the organization's goals (pGg) as well as *at least a certain percentage* of the (total of) individual's goals (pGi) realized.

In other words, an effective administrator would be a person who strives successfully to accomplish the organization's goals to the greatest possible extent, while at the same time giving adequate or ample consideration to what percentage of the goals held by individual employees is achieved. At this point, then, the concept of managerial effectiveness (Me) is added to our ongoing equation as that percentage (p) of the organization's and the (total of) individuals' goals that are realized.

> (**Note:** Initially, the percentage of an individual's goals achieved would be a collective percentage; however, where individual goal achievement exists with a differentiated reward system and a varying pay scale exists, the effectiveness of any one person could be evaluated as well.)

Thus

$$Me = (pGg) + (pGi)$$

Similarly, if we accept that managerial acts (Aplanning, Aorganizing, Astaffing, etc.) are a function of a percentage (% of the attainment of) of Gg and Gi, then

$$M = F\ (<pGg + (pGi>)$$

Further, if G (Gg + Gi) is known, it follows that Gi) is a function of it.

> (**Note:** For those interested, a much more detailed analysis of this mathematical model seeking to explain the administrative process is available in Zeigler and Bowie, 1995, pp. 115-120.)

(See Figure 3 below)

Figure 3

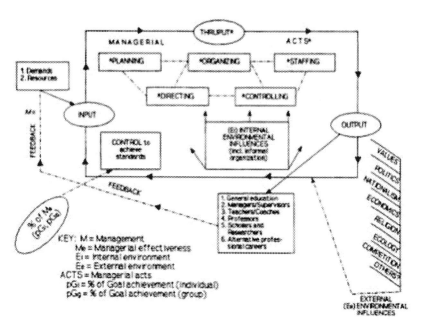

A System Analysis Model for Managerial Effectiveness
in a Professional Preparation Program for
Development Physical Activity Administrators

Coordinating Systems Analysis with Human and Natural Ecologic Interaction in the *Personal* Development of the Administrator

But what of *the individual* who is involved professionally in the managerial task itself--i.e., the first-level, second-level, etc. administrator? Adoption of this approach mandates that this person should have regular opportunities for *both* personal and professional growth. This can be accomplished by implementing a similar plan for the administrator, also, one that outlines a system analysis of the administrator's own human ecologic interaction as he or she strives *to achieve a life purpose in this profession* while concurrently serving the organization's clientele and the larger community.

If this is to be carried out successfully, such a plan should also be based on a model that includes (1) *input* factors such as demands and resources; (2) *thruput* factors such as planning, evaluation, general & professional education, and evaluation; (3)

tangible *output* factors such as (possibly) raising a family, professional achievement, and community service, and (4) intangible *user goals'* factors such as emotional maturity, personal and social fulfillment, homeostasis and self-regulation, health & fitness, and personal & social value realization.

Basically, the discussion at this point outlines how physical activity administrators can use a systems analysis approach to achieve optimal health (so-called wellness) for an effective personal and professional life within a reasonably balanced lifestyle. The idea of achieving optimal health within one's lifestyle has been equated with, and compressed in recent years by many to, the concept of "wellness":

> Wellness can be described as a lifestyle designed to reach one's highest potential for wholeness and wellbeing. Wellness has to do with a zest for living, feeling good about oneself, having goals and purposes for life . . . This concept is far more than freedom from symptoms of illness and basic health maintenance, but reaches beyond to an optimal level of well-being (*ERIC Digest* 3, 1986).

These thoughts and ideas are really not new, but they have been placed in a more modern perspective here. Many years ago Jesse Feiring Williams defined positive health as "the ability to live best and serve most." The wellness movement has similarly recommended a balanced lifestyle. It has encouraged people to assume more responsibility for their health and to view health in the same light as Williams did earlier--that is, in a positive light in which the person's "wellness" involved all aspects of a unified organism.

In this light, at the input stage the physical education and sport administrator will typically acquire a better understanding of the *demands* (e.g., required education) made upon him or her, as well as an understanding of the *resources* (e.g., genetic endowment) necessary for a satisfactory response. (See the left section of Figure 3.)

Next, at what is called the thruput stage, the manager will appreciate more fully what steps should be taken as the individual plans, organizes, and carries out life plans. At this stage these steps should be carried out optimally through self-direction with evaluation at several strategic points along the way. (See the middle section toward the top of Figure 3.)

While all of this is taking place, there are a number of external, natural and social environmental influences impinging upon the manager's development (e.g., changing societal values, declining economic status; see bottom right of Figure 3.) An administrator may have control over some of these influences, but others are often beyond control. These include both favorable and unfavorable ecologic factors. (See top right and left of Figure 3.) In the final analysis, the administrator must make a number of crucial decisions throughout life. Such decisions may be made before the fact, so to speak, while others are made as best possible in response to natural and social factors that may often be completely or partially beyond the manager's ability to control them.

In the third or output stage of an administrator's life viewed through a system analysis perspective, the manager will be asked to consider what she or he wants both her/his extrinsic, measurable and her/his intrinsic, non-measurable life goals to be. The administrator will need also to seek some sort of relationship between these measurable goals and what may be called intrinsic (i.e., typically less measurable life goals).

(**Note:** See "tangible" output at right of
Figure 3 and "intangible" output stated
as "user goals" at the bottom left of
Figure 3.)

In the first case, the tangible output, this refers to the person's achievement in his or her chosen career or occupation, as well as family life (however defined) and community service. In the second instance, he or she will need to assess the matter of achievement of personal and social fulfillment through the possible self-realization of those values that are felt to be most important.

Finally, toward the end of this system loop, provision should be made for feedback resulting in advice to the next generation. This lifelong process for the individual is typically influenced by (1) such *external environmental influences* as (e.g.) the economic status of the society; (2) such favorable ecologic factors as (e.g.) adequate medical care; and (3) such unfavorable ecologic factors as (e.g.) the presence of noxious agents & hazards.

Merging the Two Approaches to Achieve
Both: A Successful Professional Life and
a Personally Fulfilling Life

Turning attention away from self-management (i.e., the personal life pattern of the individual physical activity administrator) and back to the overall organizational administrative task itself, it becomes apparent that these two managerial techniques can be merged successfully. Whether these techniques will be in any particular organization involved with the administration of sport and physical activity depends on the overall administrative philosophy prevailing. On the surface an ecological orientation merged with a systems analysis approach to management would almost necessarily result in an "organizational management climate" that is eclectic in nature.

An "eclectic" administrative style may be needed because of the increasing number of situations today where a managerial team is responsible for the direction in which the organization is heading. This means that it may include, where possible and when desirable, any or all aspects of the traditional, behavioral, or decision-making patterns of administrative behavior. Thus administrators may find themselves functioning with an amalgam of traditional principles, cooperative behavioralist ideas, and decisionalist competitive strategies (Gibson, Ivancevich, and Donnelly, 1997, pp. 433-439).

Conclusion

In the twenty-first century, such an "amalgamated" approach to professional *and* personal management behavior as discussed here may indeed become both necessary and desirable. This would be true so long as the original formulation of aims and objectives has occurred democratically. And, as it has happened, in Western culture people have been increasingly involved in the decision-making process in all aspects of life. As a result, an organization that fails to prepare its people adequately (i.e., both theoretically and emotionally) for the introduction of change could well find its seemingly realizable goals to be thwarted--or at least temporarily blocked--by (1) human conflicts, (2) natural or cultural barriers within the general (external), or (3) changing interpersonal and/or situational circumstances within the immediate (internal) environment (Mikalachki, A., Zeigler, E.F., & Leyshon, G.A., 1988, pp. 1-17).

In respect to the organization itself and its achievement of predetermined group and individual goals, it should be borne in mind that such organizational "growth" does not necessarily mean growth in size. This is especially important where an "ecological-oriented" business strategy has been adopted on the basis of an overall philosophical stance. It does mean that the adaptive behavior of those involved in the administrative task who (1) subscribe to an "ecological orientation" philosophically and (2) employ a systems approach functionally should be in a strong position to help the organization to remain viable, to be stronger, to remain competitive, and to be increasingly more effective and efficient in the accomplishment of its long range aims and immediately realizable objectives.

Finally, similar problems or obstacles of varying nature and intensity may arise within the broader general (external) environment. Of course, the hope is that such situations would serve as challenges to physical activity administrators and their teams. The response to problems or obstacles should be heuristic in nature in the sense that a particular management team would be prepared to react to the prevailing demands and needs by adapting or possible adjusting means, behavior, and even ends at some point along the line. Developmental physical activity administrators should proceed only on the basis that the future belongs to those who manage effectively and efficiently in the pursuit of planned organizational goals.

References

Bayles, M.D. (1981). *Professional Ethics*. Belmont, CA: Wadsworth.

Epstein, J. (1997). Rio Summit's promises still unfulfilled. *The Globe and Mail* (Toronto), March 13, A12.

George, C.S. (1972). *The history of management thought (2nd Ed.)*. Englewood Cliffs, NJ: Prentice-Hall.

Gibson, J.I., Ivancevich, J.M., & Donnelly, J.H., Jr. (1997). *Organizations (9th Ed.)*. Chicago, IL: Irwin.

Hawley, A.H. (1986). *Human ecology: A theoretical essay*. Chicago: Univ. of Chicago Press.

Katz, R.L. (Sept.-Oct. 1974). Skills of an effective administrator. *Harvard Business Review*, **51**, 5:90-112.

Mackenzie, R.A. (1969). The management process in 3-D. *Harvard Education Review*, **47**: 80-87.

Mikalachki, A,, Zeigler, E.F., & Leyshon, G.A. (1988). *Change process in sport and physical education management*. Champaign, IL: Stipes.

Milstein, M.M. & Belasco, J.A. (1973). *Educational administration and the behavioral sciences: A systems perspective*. Boston: Allyn.

Prevention (July 1988). High health in the middle years. **40**: 7: 35-36, 38-47, 100, 105-107, 110.

Zeigler, E.F. (1964). *Philosophical foundations for physical, health, and recreation education*. Englewood Cliffs, NJ: Prentice-Hall.

Zeigler, E.F. (1989). *An introduction to sport and physical philosophy*. Carmel, IN: Benchmark Press.

Zeigler, E.F. (1992). *Professional ethics for sport managers*. Champaign, IL: Stipes.

Zeigler, E. F. (2003). *Socio-Cultural Foundations of Physical Education and Educational Sport*. Aachen, Germany: Meyer and Meyer.

Zeigler, E.F. & Bowie, G.W. (2007) *Management competency development in sport and physical education*. Victoria, BC: Trafford.